AF385724

Current Topics in Pathology

Ergebnisse der Pathologie

Edited by

E. Grundmann · **W. H. Kirsten**
Münster   *Chicago*

Advisory Board

Volume 58

With 69 Figures

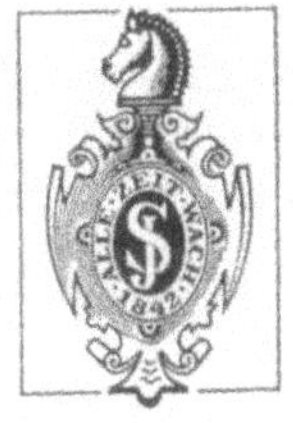

Springer-Verlag   Berlin · Heidelberg · New York   1973

ISBN-13: 978-3-642-65686-6   e-ISBN-13: 978-3-642-65684-2
DOI: 10.1007/978-3-642-65684-2

Typesetting, printing and binding: Universitätsdruckerei H. Stürtz AG, Würzburg

Contents

List of Contributors

GÜNTER DELLING, Pathologisches Institut der Universität, Martinistraße 52, D-2000 Hamburg-20, Germany

GÖTZ FREYTAG, Pathologisches Institut der Universität, Martinistraße 52, D-2000 Hamburg-20, Germany

O. KLINGE, Pathologisches Institut der Universität, Josef-Schneider-Straße 2, D-8700 Würzburg, Germany

GÜNTER KLÖPPEL, Pathologisches Institut der Universität, Martinistraße 52, D-2000 Hamburg-20, Germany

GISELA MOLZ, Anatomisches Institut der Universität, Gloriastraße 19, CH-8006 Zürich, Switzerland

U. N. RIEDE, Pathologisches Institut der Universität, Schönbeinstraße 40, CH-4056 Basel, Switzerland

HANSPETER ROHR, Pathologisches Institut der Universität, Schönbeinstraße 40, CH-4056 Basel, Switzerland

From the Department of Pathology, University of Basle, Switzerland

Experimental Metabolic Disorders and the Subcellular Reaction Pattern*

(Morphometric Analysis of Hepatocyte Mitochondria)

H. P. ROHR and U. N. RIEDE

With 25 Figures

Contents

I. Introduction

Disease is not the imposition of new, different structures and functions but simply the quantitative alteration—increase or decrease—of existing pathways. This concept, established by FORBUS (1943), ist still valid today, for the repertory of alterations is sharply limited, and usually a great many agents act through a common morphologic pathway. Up to now, only a

---

* Dedicated to Prof. Dr. med. H. U. Zollinger on the occasion of his sixtieth birthday

few attempts have been made to investigate such cellular reactions (Trump et al., 1971). The quantitative analysis of ultrastructural changes in injured cells is one of the premises to characterize the patterns of cellular reaction. Such a quantitation is even more important, if fruitful co-operation with other branches of science is aspired to.

The present study was undertaken to compose the different quantitative changes of injured hepatocytes in a reaction pattern. It is focused on mitochondria, and thus constitutes an approach to a quantitative pathology of cell organelles.

II. Principles of Morphometry

Like stereology, morphometric work is based on principles of integral geometry. In morphometry measurements are reduced to counting processes, whereby rigorous random sampling is essential at all stages: from the choice of the animals, to the selection of tissue blocks up to the sampling and analysis of the electron micrographs at different magnifications.

Morphometric results are mean values and therefore their validity must be tested by statistical methods.

Morphometric methods render possible
—Estimation of volumes
—Estimation of surfaces
—Estimation of number of structures

Terminology and symbols (for details see also Weibel 1969):

In morphometry double symbols are used: The first capital letter defines the parameter and the second capital letter the reference system (i. e. the cell component or cell organelle)

V	Volume of structure	cm^3
A	Area of structure	cm^2
N	Number of structure	cm°
S	Surface of structure	cm^2
VV	Volume density of structures in tissue	cm^3/cm^3
AA	Area density of structures in tissue	cm^2/cm^2
SV	Surface density of structures in tissue	m^2/cm^3
NV	Numerical density of structures in tissue	cm^{-3}

1. Morphometric Principles for Estimating Volumes

By further development of the so-called Delesse-principle (AA = VV) the Russian geologist Glagoleff proved that AA could also be estimated by counting the test points (PP) of regular point lattice superimposed on the section. The fraction of all points enclosed by a cell structure (PP) is equal to AA, VV respectively (Fig. 1). In a nutshell, estimation of the volume density (VV) of a cell structure can be done by estimating the area fraction or the point fraction.

2. Morphometric Principles for Estimating Surfaces

The surface density SV of a distinct cell structure is directly derived from counts of the intersection points I of the surface contour of profiles with test lines of known length LT.

From these relations (Fig. 2) the following equation can be drawn:

$$SV = 2 \cdot I/LT$$

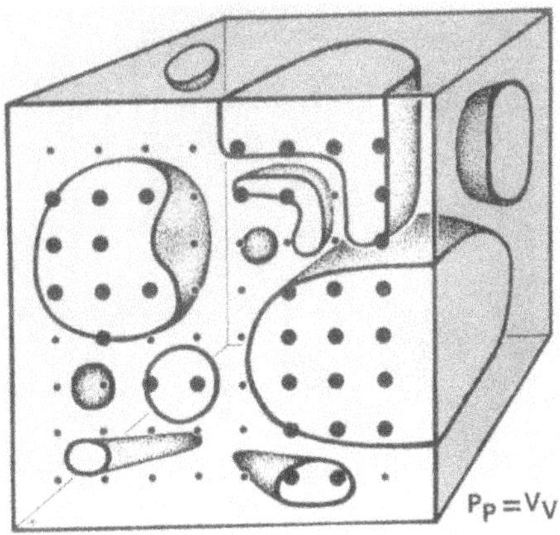

Fig. 1. Diagrammatic representation of the GLAGOLEFF principle

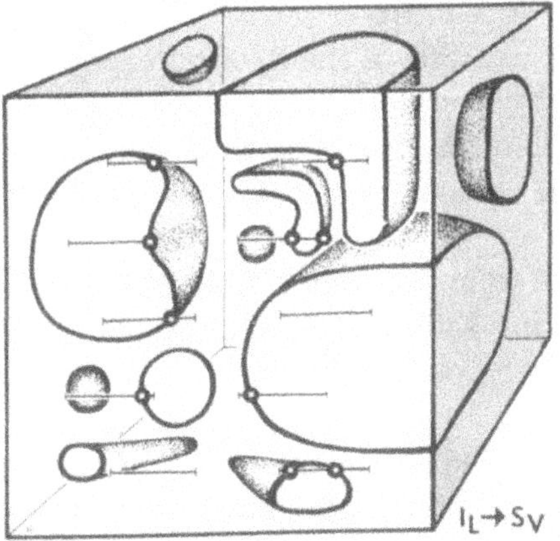

Fig. 2. Diagrammatic representation of the stereologic principle for surface estimation

3. Methods for Determining the Number of Structures

The numerical density of structures per unit volume (NV), which can be estimated from the average number of profiles of a distinct cell structure per unit area in sections (Fig. 3), depends on the shape and size of the structures in question.

1*

A useful method for the estimation of the numerical density has been developed by Weibel and Gomez (1962):

$$NV = \frac{K}{\beta} \cdot \frac{NA^{3/2}}{VV^{1/2}}$$

where the coefficient β relates to shape and K to the size distribution.

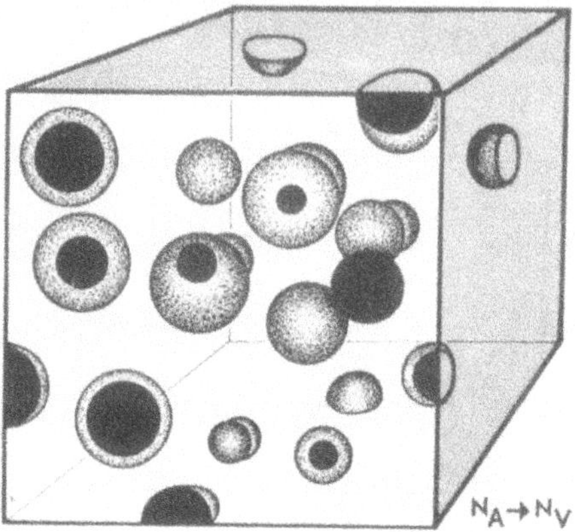

Fig. 3. Diagrammatic representation of the relation between the number of structures in area and volume

III. Morphometric Procedure

For a morphometric analysis of the liver parenchyma standardized experimental conditions are indispensable.

— If possible, sacrificing of the animals at the same time of day. In this way, the typical circadian changes of hepatocytes can be avoided (Rohr et al., 1969).

— Biopsy of liver tissue from the right liver lobe.

— Use of the same fixing solution. S-collidine—buffered OsO_4 proved to be most appropriate for the observation of the smooth endoplasmic reticulum (Rohr et al., 1970).

— In all experiments we studied the morphometric parameters of the middle part of the liver lobule, since mitochondria in this field show especially homogeneous shapes (Riede and Rohr, 1971; Stulz, 1972; Reith et al., 1969).

Because of the wide range of cell structures we used a modified method of multiple-stage sampling according to Weibel (1969), Weibel et al. (1969a, b), Rohr et al. (1971).

Stage I. 5 randomly-sampled liver tissue blocks were cut semithin, and 10 test areas were evaluated at 1000 × magnification using an automatic sampling stage microscope (Wild; Heerbrugg, Switzerland).

At this stage, the volume density of hepatocyte nuclei and extralobular space, and the numerical density of hepatocellular nuclei were evaluated.

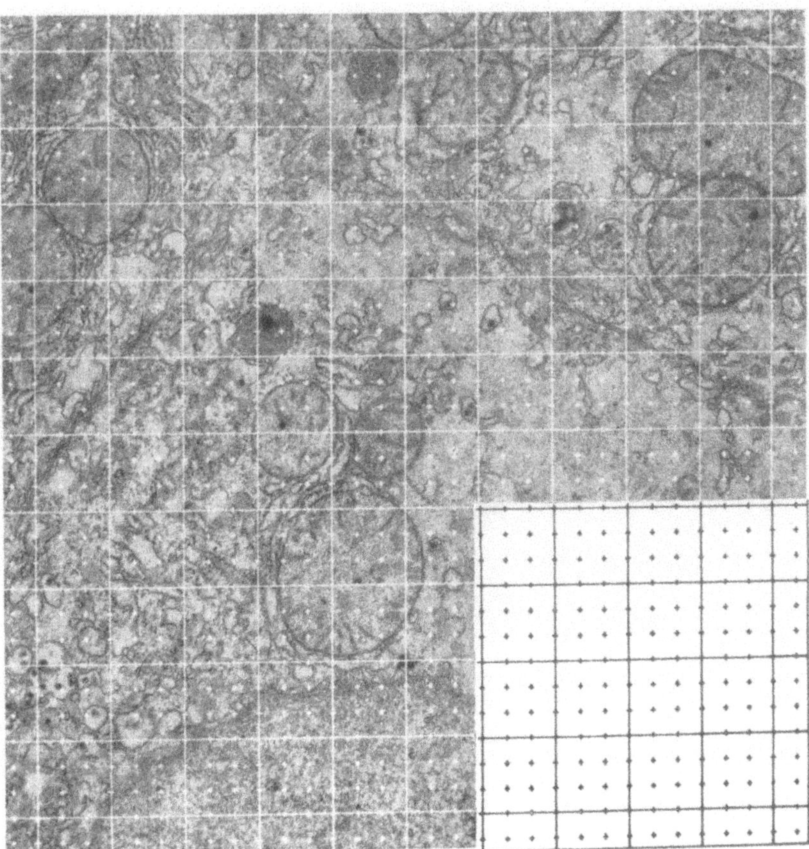

Fig. 4. Double lattice test system superimposed on section of a hepatocyte. (Stage II of morphometric analysis). 2 × 5000 ×

Stage II. From 3 blocks ultrathin sections were cut for electron microscopy. By systematic random sampling, 6 electron micrographs per block were taken at 5000 × magnification.

Morphometric evaluation was done with a 9:1 double lattice test-screen, either by projecting the micrographs onto the test screen of a projector (final magnification: 45000 ×) or by enlarging the micrographs together with the double test lattice (final magnification: 15000 ×) (Fig. 4).

At this level, the volume densities of the following cell components were determined: Nuclei, extrahepatocellular space, cytoplasm, mitochondria, lysosomes and microbodies. For the last two the fine mesh of the test screen was used. Furthermore, the numerical densities of mitochondria and microbodies were calculated from the corresponding values.

Stage III. Finally, 6 micrographs of each of the 3 blocks were taken at primary magnification of 10000× by analogous rigorous random sampling. Morphometric analysis was done by using a multipurpose test screen (WEIBEL, 1969) with 50 lines (Fig. 5).

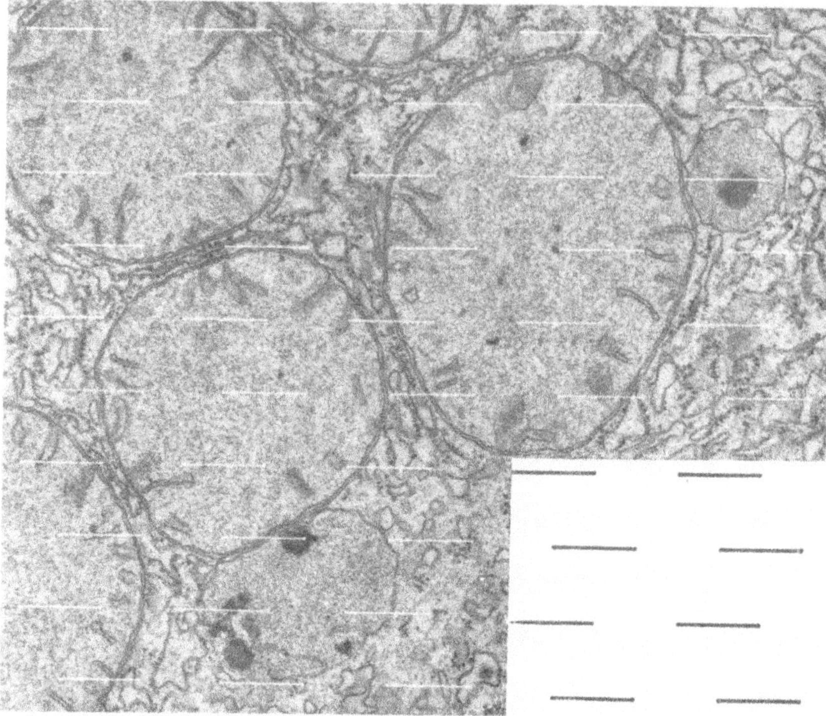

Fig. 5. Multi-purpose test screen (Weibel, 1969) superimposed on section of a hepatocyte
(Stage III of morphometric analysis). 2 × 10000 ×

At this stage, the volume densities of the remaining cell organelles and
components, the surface densities of the rough and smooth endoplasmic reticulum, the mitochondrial envelope and cristae were calculated.

In order to relate these values to the whole liver, all data were multiplied
by correcting factors:

At each stage, certain histological or cytologic structures were deliberately
not covered, such as, at 10000 × magnification, cell nuclei. Proportional to
the frequency (the volume share respectively) of these neglected structures,
in the whole liver tissue a constant error is introduced, which is balanced by
the so-called correcting factors. In this way, the morphometric values of the
individual cell compartments and the real values are adapted.

IV. Morphometric Characterization of Normal Hepatocytes

1. Primary Parameters

The hepatocyte as an entity:

Volume densities (VV):

VV EX   Extrahepatocellular space
VV H   Hepatocyte

VV NH   Nuclei
VV C   Cytoplasm

Numerical density:

NV NH   Nuclei

Cell organellae and components:

Volume densities (VV, cm^0):

VV M   Mitochondria
VV MB   Microbodies
VV SER   Smooth endoplasmic reticulum
VV RER   Rough endoplasmic reticulum
VV F   Fat droplets
VV GF   Golgi apparatus
VV GLYCO   Glycogen
VV RIBO   Ribosomal area (i. e. free ribosomes)
VV LY   Lysosomes
VV G   Cytoplasmic ground substance (= hyaloplasm)

Numerical densities (NV, cm^{-3}):

NV M   Mitochondria
NV MB   Microbodies

Surface densities (SV, m^2/cm^3):

SV RER   Rough endoplasmic reticulum
SV SER   Smooth endoplasmic reticulum
SV MO   Mitochondrial outer membranes
SV MC   Mitochondrial inner membranes (cristae resp.).

2. Secondary Parameters

For characterization of the liver cell as a functional unit the values of the primary parameters must be converted and expressed e. g. in volume densities per unit volume hepatocyte, cytoplasm, or in absolute values such as mean volume of a single mitochondrion, number of mitochondria per hepatocyte.

These simple combinations of primary parameters are called secondary parameters.

List of secondary parameters

The hepatocytes as an entity:

VVH/NVNH   Single volume of a 'mononuclear' hepatocyte
VVC/NVNH   Absolute volume of cytoplasm per hepatocyte
VVC/VVH   Volume of cytoplasm per unit volume hepatocyte
VVNH/NVNH   Single volume of liver cell nucleus
VVNH/VVH   Volume of nuclei per unit volume hepatocyte

Cell components

Volumes

VVCOMP/NVNH	Absolute volume of a component per hepatocyte
VVCOMP/VVH	Volume of a component per unit volume hepatocyte
VVCOMP/VVC	Volume of a component per unit volume cytoplasm

Surfaces

SVCOMP/NVNH	Surface of a component per hepatocyte
SVCOMP/VVH	Surface of a component per unit volume hepatocyte
SVCOMP/VVC	Surface of a component per unit volume cytoplasm
SVCOMP/VVCOMP	Surface of a component per unit volume component

In general, the surface densities of the following cell components are evaluated: RER

SER

MO, MC

Number of Components

NVCOMP/NVNH	Number of component per hepatocyte
NVCOMP/VVH	Number of a component per unit volume hepatocyte
NVCOMP/VVC	Number of a component per unit volume cytoplasm

The numerical densities of liver cell nuclei, mitochondria and microbodies were evaluated.

Mean Single Volume of Organelles

(Considering shape correcting factors, e. g., VVM/NVM single volume of a mitochondrion).

The mitochondrial shape in the hepatocytes varies considerably (Reith *et al.*, 1970). However, since the mitochondrial shape is inserted as a factor in the formula for the calculation of the numerical density, developed by Weibel and Gomez (1963), the values of the mitochondrial single volume, calculated from the quotient VVM/NVM, must be considered estimated values. For these reasons, we calculated the mitochondrial single volume also from the surface (SVMO) - volume (VVM) ratio. Although in this calculation the shape factor has no effect, comparative values were obtained. In consequence, the determination of the quotient VVM/NVM is sufficient for the calculation of the mitochondrial single volume of the middle part of the liver lobules.

Surfaces of Cell Components

e. g.: Mitochondria

SVMO/NVM	Surface of mitochondrial outer membrane per single mitochondrion
SVMC/NVM	Surface of mitochondrial cristae per single mitochondrion

Numerical Proportions

e. g.: NVM/NVMB   Number of mitochondria per microbody.

The evaluation of the cellular morphometric data and statistics (Student's t-test) was performed with a "multipurpose" morphometric program (ROHR and KELLER, 1972), using an Olivetti computer system Programma 602.

The *Multipurpose-Morphometric-Computer-Program (MMCP)* allows an *almost fully automated evaluation* of light microscopic and ultrastructural morphometric analyses. This program was developed for the OLIVETTI PROGRAMMA 602 Computer System, consisting of an Olivetti Programma 602, a magnetic tape unit MLU 600 and a terminal TE 318. The MMCP is organized according to the modular concept so that individual program items can be applied separately. Due to this fact, the MMCP can be adapted to any morphometric evaluation system and used for the morphometric analysis of all organs and tissues in light and electron microscopy. Basically, the MMCP is organized in the following way: The *first step* consists in the *evaluation of the mean values* (primary parameters) and *significance* (Student's t-test, F-test) of the counting data. As a *second step*, the *secondary parameters* can be calculated from the primary ones. The *third step* provides the possibility of comprising the values of the primary parameters in *arbitrary groups* and of converting them again into corresponding secondary parameters. The calculation of the primary and secondary parameters of the groups is followed again by the evaluation of their significance.

V. Quantitative Changes of Hepatic Mitochondria under Experimental Conditions

1. Definition and Morphometric Characterization of the Most Important Changes in Liver Mitochondria

Mitochondrial Proliferation. By mitochondrial proliferation we mean the numerical increase of mitochondria per hepatocyte. This means that the mitochondrial volume density and the absolute volume of mitochondria per hepatocyte are increased. The mitochondrial single volume may (but need not) remain unchanged. However, under numerous experimental conditions, a process of mitochondrial proliferation can be observed where the number of mitochondria per hepatocyte increases, the absolute volume of mitochondria per hepatocyte usually remains constant, but where the mitochondrial single volume is drastically reduced.

In the following, this kind of proliferation is referred to as incomplete proliferation and has to be distinguished from complete proliferation.

Enlargement of the Mitochondrial Single Volume. As a general principle, the mitochondrial single volume can be enlarged by disturbed mitochondrial division, mitochondrial growth or swelling processes. The last two processes can be differentiated morphometrically.

Table 1a. Experimental design

Experiment	Dosage of applied drugs	Form of application	Observation period	Animals and tissue analysed:
1. Cycloheximide Inhibition of ribosomal Protein-synthesis (Actidione, Upjohn-Chicago)	3,3 mg/kg b.w.	i.p.	3, 6, 12, 48 hours after the single injection	liver of male Wistar rats weighing 180 g
2. Chloromycetin Inhibiton of mitochondrial	1800 mg/kg b.w.	i.m.	3, 6 hours after single injection	liver of male Wistar rats weighing 240 g
Proteinsynthesis (Synthomycetin, LePetit-Milano)	1000 mg/kg b.w. daily	i.p.	after 5 days of application	liver of male Wistar rats weighing 250 g
3. Folic acid (Fluka-Buchs, No. 460035)	250 mg/kg b.w.	i.v.	6, 12, 24 hours after the single injection	liver of male Wistar rats weighing 195 g
4. Malonic acid Inhibition of succinate dehydrogenase (Fluka-Buchs, No. 63290)	250 mg/kg b.w.	i.p.	3, 6, 12, 24 hours after the single injection	liver of male Wistar rats weighing 210 g
5. Orotic acid Inhibition of Purine-nucleotide synthesis	1 % added to a semi-synthetic diet (WOOLEY and SEBRELL, 1945)	p.o.	after 3, 5, 7 days of application	liver of male Wistar rats weighing 200 g
6. Vitamin-E deficiency lack of biologic antioxidans	diet rich in carbohydrates and deficient in Vit. E. (SCHWYTER et al., 1967)	p.o.	9 month after feeding the diet	liver of male Wistar rats initial weight 100 g terminal weight 360 g

Table 1a (Continued)

Experiment	Dosage of applied drugs	Form of application	Observation period	Animals and tissue analysed:
7. D-penicillamine copper-deficiency (Distamine, Dista-Liverpool)	200 mg/kg b.w.	p.o.	after 7 weeks of application	liver of male Wistar-rats initial weight 100 g terminal weight 150 g
8. Riboflavin-deficiency lack of prosthetic group of mitochondrial dehydrogenases	diet deficient in riboflavin (TANDLER et al., 1968)	p.o.	after 3, 14, 18, 42 days after feeding the diet	liver of male Swiss mice initial weight 18 g terminal weight 12 g
9. $^2/_3$ hepatectomia Liver-regeneration (ref. HIGGINS and ANDERSON, 1931)	1000 µC ^{3}H-thymidine 24 hours postop.	i.p.	40 Min., 6, 12, 24, 48, 96 hours after the single injection	labeled hepatocytes of male Wistar rats weighing 160 g
10. Hepatocytes in the perinatal period (ref. ROHR et al., 1971)	—	—	3 days before birth	liver of male fetuses of Wistar rats
			1, 3, 8 days after delivery	liver of newborn male Wistar rats
11. Starvation and refeeding	—	—	3, 6, 9 days of starvation	liver of male Wistar rats initial weight 240 g terminal weight 120 g
			3 days after refeeding of starved rats during 9 days	liver of male Wistar rats initial weight 120 g terminal weight 150 g

In the case of *mitochondrial growth*, the mitochondrial single volume increases, the number of mitochondria per hepatocyte may (but need not) remain constant, and the surface of mitochondrial cristae per unit volume mitochondrion is not reduced.

In the case of a *mitochondrial swelling process*, the mitochondrial single volume also increases, but the surface of mitochondrial cristae per unit volume mitochondrion is reduced (Fig. 19). The number of mitochondria per hepatocyte is reduced in most cases.

Mitochondrial swelling is usually characterized by the fact that the mitochondrial matrix is eluted (matricolysis) and, therefore, appears more translucent in the electron microscope. At the same time, mitochondrial cristae are reduced due to cristolysis. However, very often matricolysis and cristolysis occur separately. The counterpart is an isolated cristae proliferation, or matrix growth.

Cristae Proliferation. In the case of cristae proliferation (Fig. 19), the surface density of the mitochondrial cristae per unit volume liver tissue (SVMC), per unit volume hepatocyte (SVMC/VVH) and, in most cases, also per unit volume mitochondrion is increased.

2. Mitochondria during Mitosis

Since the first light microscopic observation of mitochondria by ALTMANN (1890), the biogenesis of mitochondria has been the subject of numerous studies. Only lately has it been possible to show by the electron microscopic observation of figures of mitochondrial division that mitochondria originate from pre-existing ones (ref. ROHR et al., 1971).

The fact that DNA and RNA were found in mitochondria (ref. KROON, 1969) leads to the conclusion that in the cell, mitochondria enjoy a certain degree of autonomy as a self-replicating system. Despite these findings, many questions have not been clarified until now. Mainly quantitative data about the reaction of mitochondria during mitosis are still lacking. To throw light upon this question, we made a combined electron microscopic-autoradiographic-morphometric analysis of the hepatocyte 24 hours after partial hepatectomia (Table 1) (ROHR et al., 1970).

40 minutes after the injection of ^{3}H-thymidine, the labeled hepatocytes do not show ultrastructural changes (Fig. 6a), except for almost total glycogen depletion. In particular, the number of lysosomes has not increased. The morphometric analysis (Table 2) shows that during the DNA synthesis phase there are no signs of hepatocytic dedifferentiation.

Whereas the single volume of hepatocytes corresponds to that of controls, the volume densities of the rough endoplasmic reticulum and the ribosomal areas are somewhat increased (ROHR et al., 1970). Therefore, the increased volume density of lysosomes, observed during the pre-regenerating phase after $^2/_3$ hepatectomia, is due to cell restructuring-processes, reflecting increased cell activity and not dedifferentiation of hepatocytes, as mentioned by BECKER and LANE (1968).

Table 1 b. Morphometric basic values of the experiments

Experiment	Observation period	Symbol	Mean value	S.e.	Symbol	Mean value	S.e.	Symbol	Mean value	S.e.
Normal rats		NANH	5.388	0.585	NAM	18.021	2.113	VVM	0.167	0.006
		IMC	6.666	0.322	IMO	21.252	1.947			
		NAMB	2.483	0.133	VVMB	0.008	0.001			
Normal mice		NANH	5.211	0.444	NAM	18.223	1.428	VVM	0.197	0.004
		NAMB	6.093	0.353	VVMB	0.009	0.0001	IMC	7.111	0.783
Normal desert rats		NANH	4.645	0.378	NAM	9.777	1.095	VVM	0.198	0.031
		NAMB	2.555	0.236	VVMB	0.005	0.0007	IMC	10.208	0.659
1. Cycloheximide	3 h	NANH	5.286	0.412	NAM	39.555	3.307	VVM	0.239	0.020
		NAMB	5.185	0.606	VVMB	0.013	0.001			
		IMC	2.087	0,405	IMO	5.204	1.392			
	6 h	NANH	4.346	0.293	NAM	39.629	2.657	VVM	0.241	0.010
		NAMB	5.629	1.796	VVMB	0.013	0.001			
		IMC	1.481	0.074	IMO	4.407	0.329			
	12 h	NANH	4.266	0.415	NAM	28.962	1.614	VVM	0.224	0.008
		NAMB	4.444	0.756	VVMB	0.011	0.0008			
		IMC	1.629	0.267	IMO	3.926	0.658			
	24 h	NANH	3.926	0.329	NAM	25.518	0.996	VVM	0.260	0.008
		NAMB	5.148	0.965	VVMB	0.011	0.0005			
		IMC	1.444	0.169	IMO	1.926	0.316			
	48 h	NANH	3.583	0.170	NAM	24.255	1.151	VVM	0.196	0.013
		NAMB	3.740	0.472	VVMB	0.010	0.002			
		IMC	0.629	0.259	IMO	1.999	0.421			
2. Chloromycetin	3 h	NANH	5.483	0.438	NAM	16.964	1.969	VVM	0.180	0.015
		IMC	12.407	1.276	IMO	14.240	1.790			
	6 h	NANH	5.706	0.425	NAM	16.870	1.677	VVM	0.203	0.019
		IMC	9.166	2.084	IMO	14.537	0.636			
	5 d	NANH	4.500	0.038	NAM	13.203	1.828	VVM	0.299	0.011
		IMC	10.901	0.410	IMO	10.311	0.431			

Table 1b (Continued)

Experiment	Observation period	Symbol	Mean value	S.e.	Symbol	Mean value	S.e.	Symbol	Mean value	S.e.
3. Folic acid	6h	NANH IMC	5.093 9.370	0.335 0.805	NAM	13.481	0.962	VVM	0.217	0.018
	12h	NANH IMC	5.113 9.143	0.013 1.065	NAM	11.407	0.880	VVM	0.215	0.004
	24h	NANH IMC	4.427 5.926	0.052 1.130	NAM	14.148	1.175	VVM	0.172	0.025
4. Malonic acid	3h	IMC	5.997	1.715				VVM	0.192	0.005
	6h	IMC	4.448	0.305				VVM	0.229	0.001
	12h	IMC	6.271	0.368				VVM	0.200	0.009
	24h	IMC	4.184	0.669				VVM	0.218	0.011
5. Orotic acid	3d	NANH IMC	4.195 5.156	0.142 0.925	NAM	21.037	1.530	VVM	0.162	0.012
	5d	NANH IMC	5.443 5.066	0.221 0.528	NAM	17.739	2.905	VVM	0.140	0.026
	7d	NANH IMC	4.553 5.947	0.601 0.882	NAM	15.481	1.650	VVM	0.186	0.011
6. Vitamin-E-deficiency	+E 9 m	NANH IMC	4.632 4.666	0.089 0.111	NAM	10.777	0.555	VVM	0.212	0.006
	—E 9 m	NANH IMC	4.485 11.111	0.053 1.345	NAM	16.208	0.759	VVM	0.261	0.012
7. D-Penicillamine	7w	IMC	8.478	0.326	NAM IMO	19.370 11.981	0.537 0.304	VVM	0.228	0.011
8. Riboflavin-deficiency	3d	NANH NAMB	3.977 6.833	0.369 0.339	NAM VVMB	15.870 0.010	0.518 0.0001	VVM IMC	0.200 8.388	0.011 1.951
	14d	NANH NAMB	5.122 5.404	0.318 1.662	NAM VVMB	14.675 0.007	1.867 0.001	VVM IMC	0.205 8.129	0.018 1.719

	28 d	NANH	7.533	0.407	NAM	13.074	0.465	VVM	0.284	0.009
		NAMB	3.759	0.048	VVMB	0.009	0.0001	IMC	9.907	0.742
	42 d	NANH	7.766	0.566	NAM	12.240	1.454	VVM	0.308	0.007
		NAMB	3.333	0.096	VVMB	0.007	0.0001	IMC	13.870	0.632
9. ²/₃ Hepatectomia	40 min	NANH	1.888	0.351	NAM	20.685	1.340	VVM	0.174	0.013
	6 h	NANH	1.293	0.199	NAM	17.928	1.272	VVM	0.161	0.014
	12 h	NANH	1.109	0.099	NAM	15.095	1.752	VVM	0.165	0.017
	24 h	NANH	1.444	0.175	NAM	19.333	3.451	VVM	0.185	0.028
	48 h	NANH	1.445	0.163	NAM	21.294	1.761	VVM	0.297	0.020
	96 h	NANH	1.748	0.271	NAM	22.315	1.463	VVM	0.273	0.019
10. Hepatocytes in the perinatal period	—3 d	NANH	9.157	0.657	NAM	16.533	0.870	VVM	0.127	0.015
	0	NANH	3.760	0.260	NAM	7.308	0.543	VVM	0.128	0.006
	+1 d	NANH	6.266	0.466	NAM	11.422	0.823	VVM	0.253	0.015
	+3 d	NANH	7.718	0.817	NAM	17.254	1.191	VVM	0.252	0.016
	+8 d	NANH	6.223	0.610	NAM	16.583	1.266	VVM	0.225	0.014
11. Starvation and refeeding	—3 d	NANH	5.241	0.312	NAM	21.388	1.001	VVM	0.417	0.031
		IMC	11.528	0.511						
	—6 d	NANH	5.493	0.403	NAM	19.147	1.225	VVM	0.436	0.030
		IMC	11.174	1.222						
	—9 d	NANH	8.283	1.091	NAM	13.203	3.065	VVM	0.563	0.051
		IMC	17.011	2.341						
	—9+3 d	NANH	4.040	0.291	NAM	12.250	1.057	VVM	0.261	0.014
		IMC	8.882	0.551						

Abbreviations: NANH = Number of hepatic nuclei per test area. NAM = Number of mitochondria per test area. VVM = Volume density of mitochondria. VVMB = Volume density of microbodies. IMC = Number of intersections of the mitochondrial cristae with the test-lines per test area. IMO = Number of intersections of the mitochondrial outer membrane with the test-lines per test area.

Table 2a. Morphometric data of rat hepatocytes during regeneration
after $^2/_3$ hepatectomy

Symbol		Intermitotic Hepatocytes	Hepatocytes during Phase of DNA-Synthesis
VVH/NVNH	Hepatocyte single volume	4800	4950 (μm^3)
VVM/VVH	Volume of mitochondria per unit volume hepatocyte	0.165	0.171 (cm^3/cm^3)
VVM/NVM	Mitochondrial single volume	0.66	0.72 (μm^3)
NVM/NVNH	Number of mitochondria per hepatocyte	1470	1350
VVRER/VVH	RER-volume per unit volume hepatocyte	0.205	0.256 (cm^3/cm^3)
VVSER/VVH	SER-volume per unit volume hepatocyte	0.143	0.115 (cm^3/cm^3)
VVGLYCO/VVH	Glycogen-volume per unit volume hepatocyte	0.177	0.089 (cm^3/cm^3)
VVGF/VVH	Golgi-field-volume per unit volume hepatocyte	0.005	0.007 (cm^3/cm^3)
VVLYSO/VVH	Lysosome-volume per unit volume hepatocyte	0.004	0.007 (cm^3/cm^3)

Table 2b. Morphometric data of normal rat hepatocyte

Component	Symbol	Mean	Dimension	Value per "mononuclear" hepatocyte	
Hepatocyte	VVH	0.81	cm^3/cm^3	5450	μm^3
Nuclei	VVNH	0.05	cm^3/cm^3	315	μm^3
	NVNH	150.10^6	cm^{-3}	1	
Cytoplasm	VVC	0.76	cm^3/cm^3	5138	μm^3
Mitochondria	VVM	0.167	cm^3/cm^3	911	μm^3
	NVM	283.10^9	cm^{-3}	1890	
single volume	VVM/NVM			0.69	μm^3
outer membrane	SVMO	1.98	m^2/cm^3	13100	μm^2
cristae	SVMC	5.18	m^2/cm^3	44400	μm^2
Microbodies	VVMB	0.007	cm^3/cm^3	48	μm^3
	NVMB	60.10^9	cm^{-3}	420	
single volume	VVMB/NVMB			0.12	μm^3

The increase of the volume densities of the rough endoplasmic reticulum
and the ribosomal areas in the pre-regenerating phase (Rohr *et al.*, 1970)
indicates an increased protein synthesis after partial hepatectomia (Muramatsu

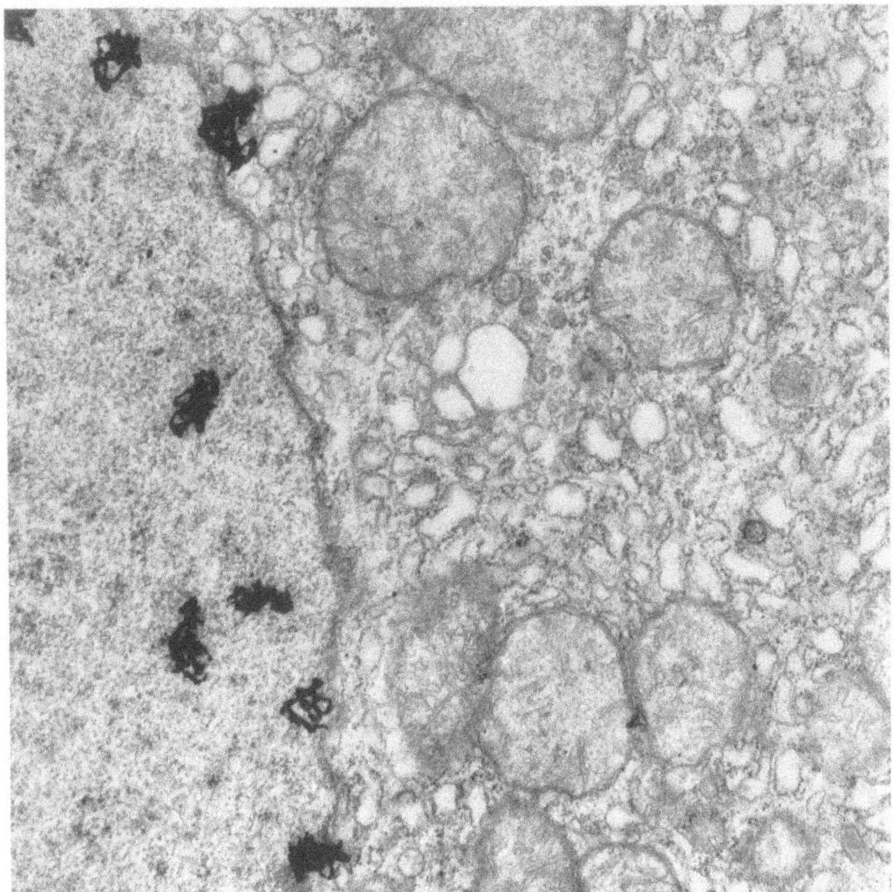

Fig. 6a. Rat hepatocyte 24 hours after partial hepatectomia and 40 minutes after a single injection of labeled thymidine. The hepatocyte with labeled nucleus does not show ultrastructural changes as compared with controls. 16000 × (electron-microscopic autoradiography)

and BUSCH, 1962; CLERICI *et al.*, 1965; TSUKADA and LIEBERMANN, 1965; MAJUMDAR *et al.*, 1967).

During the DNA-synthesis phase, the chondrioma corresponds numerically and volumetrically to that of controls (Table 2). These morphometric-autoradiographic findings show that dedifferentiation need not always precede the mitosis of facultatively postmitotic cells, e. g. of hepatocytes.

24 and 48 hours after the injection of ^{3}H-thymidine, however, the number of mitochondria per hepatocyte has decreased by 50% (Fig. 6b), whereas the mitochondrial single volume has doubled (Fig. 6c). The volume of mitochondria per hepatocyte remains unchanged (Fig. 6d). 96 hours after the injection of ^{3}H-thymidine, hepatocytes are characterized again by the original number of mitochondria per cell, and the single volumes of mitochondria are back to normal (Fig. 6b and c). These morphometric-autoradiographic find-

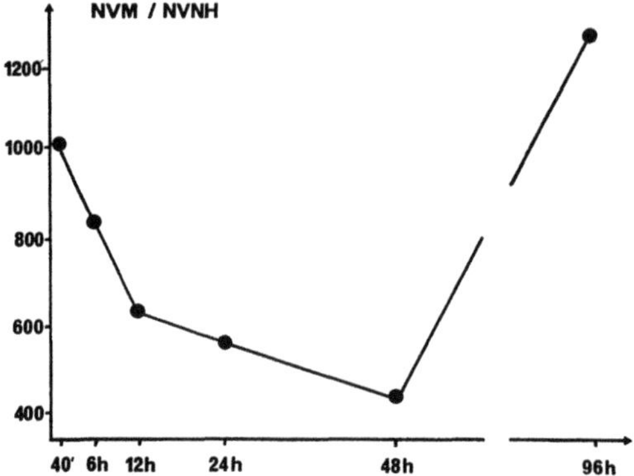

Fig. 6b. Number of mitochondria per hepatocyte (NVM/NVNH) 40 minutes—96 hours after the injection of labeled thymidine and 24–120 hours after the partial hepatectomia

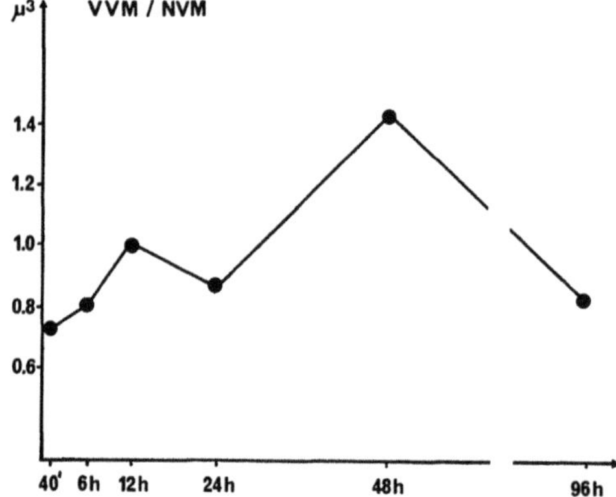

Fig. 6c. Mitochondrial single volume (VVM/NVM) 40 minutes—96 hours after the injection of labeled thymidine and 24–120 hours after the partial hepatectomia

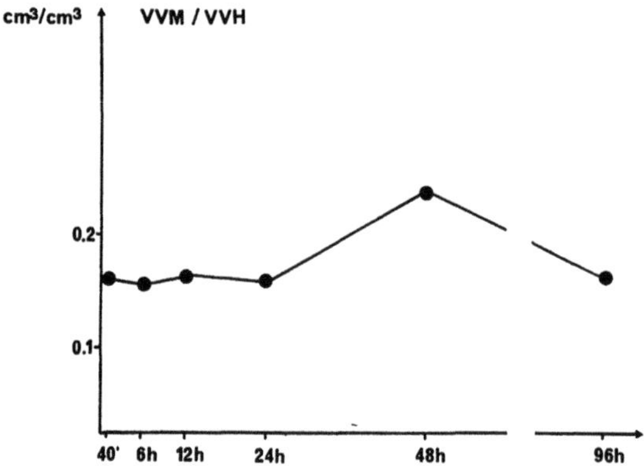

Fig. 6d. Mitochondrial volume per unit volume hepatocyte (VVM/VVH) 40 minutes — 96 hours after the injection of labeled thymidine and 24–120 hours after the partial hepatectomia

ings allow the conclusion that mitosis is followed by the division of mito-chondria.

Similar results were gained from the morphometric analysis of hepatocytes during the perinatal phase (Table 1) (ROHR *et al.*, 1971). Thereby it became clear that a first peak of mitotic activity is reached between hour 24 and 72 post partum. The cell volume has decreased by 50 %, and the number of mitochondria per cell diminished slightly. Therefore, also in this case, it may be assumed that mitochondria divide in the course of mitosis and thus safe-guard a constant mitochondrial stock of the cell.

Numerous mitochondrial division figures could be shown during the most intensive mitotic activity of hepatocytes post partum. What is striking in this connection is the fact that 24 hours post partum, i. e. at a time when at least a third of all hepatocytes has divided once, the mitochondrial single volume shows a clear increase and the mitochondrial number per cell a slight decrease. Therefore, we assume that in mitosis two daughter cells with 50 % of the mito-chondrial stock originate first. Shortly after mitosis the mitochondrial single volumes double. Due to the following division, the initial number of mito-chondria per cell and the initial mitochondrial single volume are reached again. As far as hepatocytes during the perinatal phase are concerned, it must, however, be assumed that in the first three postpartal days there is a division of at least $^1/_6$ of the mitochondria in the interphasic hepatocytes so that the number of mitochondria per cell increases to about 400 (ROHR *et al.*, 1971).

In other cell systems, e. g. Saccharomyces lactis or Chang liver cells syn-chronized by cold shock, it could be shown that mitochondrial DNA-synthesis occured at a time different from that at which nuclear DNA was synthesized (ref. MADREITER *et al.*, 1972). Furthermore, autoradiographic studies on Tetrahymena pyriformis revealed analogous results. These findings fit well with the hypothesis based on morphometric results according to which the mitochondrial division of hepatocytes follows mitosis after about 48 hours (ROHR *et al.*, 1971). MADREITER *et al.* (1972) studied this problem in a system of mechanically synchronized mouse fibroblasts (L-cells). Throughout all phases of the mitotic cycle, incorporation of ^{3}H-thymidine into mitochondrial DNA could be observed. In the early S-phase, a sixfold increase of ^{3}H-thymi-dine incorporation could be encountered, as compared with the incorporation in the G_1-phase.

Hepatic mitochondria divide not only immediately after the mitotic cycle but also during the intermitotic phase. Turnover studies of labeled precursors of mitochondrial membranes revealed a half-life for mitochondrial proteins ranging from 8.5–12.4 days (FLETSCHER and SANADI, 1961). On the basis of a quantitative-autoradiographic study, BERGERON and DROZ (1969) calculated a half-life for mitochondrial proteins amounting to 9.4 days. Assuming a mean mitochondrial number of 1600 per hepatocyte, about 80–100 mitochondria should divide daily. This explains that mitochondrial division figures are found only in very few normal intermitotic hepatocytes. Therefore, mitochondrial division figures indicate increased mitochondrial division activity.

3. Mitochondrial Proliferation

Under numerous experimental conditions, complete proliferation of mitochondria can be observed morphometrically. This kind of proliferation occurs often in cases where the cell metabolism is stimulated, such as:

1. in the regenerating phase after partial hepatectomia (Rohr et al., 1970)

2. during the postpartal period (Rohr et al., 1971)

3. in the adaptive phase after purine-biosynthesis inhibited by exogenous adenine (Riede et al., 1971)

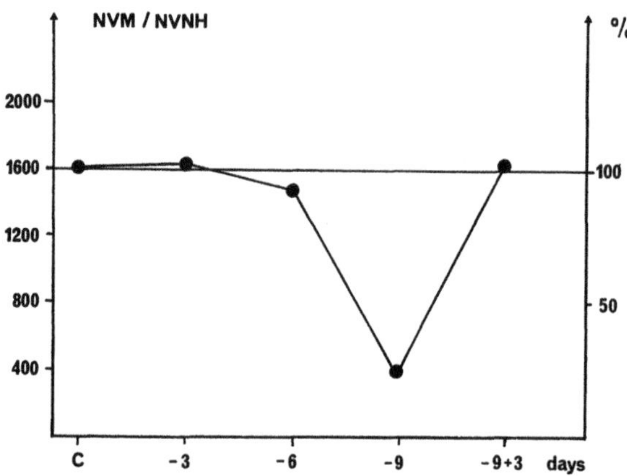

Fig. 7 a. Number of mitochondria per rat hepatocyte (NVM/NVNH) during starvation (–3, –6, –9) and refeeding (–9 +3). *C* Control rats

4. glycogen-mobilization by glucagon (Rohr et al., 1971)

5. in the recovery-phase during refeeding of starved rats (Rohr, et al., 1973).

A 9-day period of starvation (Table 1) leads to a drastic reduction of the number of mitochondria per hepatocyte, which during a 3-day refeeding period is normalized again by intensive mitochondrial proliferation (Fig. 7a and 7b). Similar results were described by Scarpelli et al. (1971), who, in addition, observed increased incorporation of labeled precursors into the DNA and membrane proteins of the hepatic mitochondria during the refeeding period. Thus, the constancy of the mitochondrial number per hepatocyte depends at least partially on adequate feeding.

In contrast to this, in the case of distinct metabolic disturbances of the liver cells in the early phase, an increase of the number of mitochondria per hepatocyte going hand in hand with a reduction of the mitochondrial single volume can be observed. An example of such a reaction pattern of the chondrioma is the inhibition of the protein synthesis by cycloheximide (Riede et al., 1971). The antibiotic cycloheximide inhibits the ribosomal protein synthesis by blocking the incorporation of amino acids as aminoacyl-transfer-RNA into the peptides (Ennis and Lubin, 1964). The mitochondrial protein synthesis, however, is not influenced by cycloheximide (Borst et al., 1967, Coggi and Scarpelli, 1970).

With respect to a single injection of cycloheximide (Table 1), the liver parenchymal cell shows a biphasic reaction (early phase: hour 3–6; late phase: hour 12–48). The early phase is characterized by a change in the morphometric parameters (Fig. 8) of mitochondria, microbodies, as well as the smooth and rough endoplasmic reticulum. In the early phase, the morphometric changes of mitochondria and microbodies are especially striking. The two cell organelles show an increase in their number per hepatocyte (Fig. 8a and c,) and numerical density. The mitochondrial single volume decreases

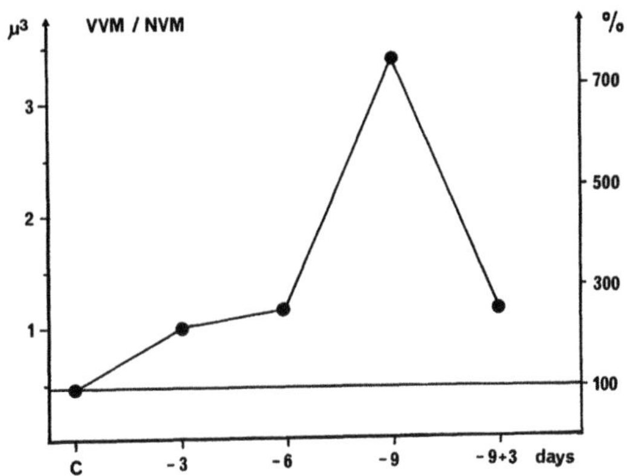

Fig. 7b. Mitochondrial single volume (VVM/NVM) of rat hepatocyte during starvation (–3, –6, –9) and refeeding (–9 +3). *C* Control rats

(Fig. 8b). In other words: Under the influence of cycloheximide, a higher number of smaller mitochondria and microbodies per hepatocyte occurs. Since in this phase the absolute volume of mitochondria per hepatocyte does not change considerably (Fig. 8e), the mitochondrial changes may be explained by division processes. As a matter of fact, numerous mitochondrial division figures are observed during this time span. The possibility of complete mitochondrial proliferation can be excluded for the following reasons:

1. 3–6 hours are too short for a synthesis of new structural proteins.

2. The incorporation of labeled leucine into the proteins of the mitochondrial outer membranes is drastically reduced by cycloheximide (SCARPELLI *et al.*, 1970).

3. In the late phase (24 and 48 hours), the surface density of the mitochondrial outer and inner membranes is reduced (Fig. 8f, g) (RIEDE *et al.*, 1971).

Such an increase in the number of mitochondria is interpreted as *incomplete* mitochondrial proliferation and must be differentiated from *complete* mitochondrial proliferation. Accordingly, the synthesis of structural proteins is inhibited, but mitochondrial division is possible despite the metabolic effects of cycloheximide. In the case of incomplete proliferation, a disturbance of the mitochondrial DNA-polymerase-system is conceivable. Thereby, the synthesis

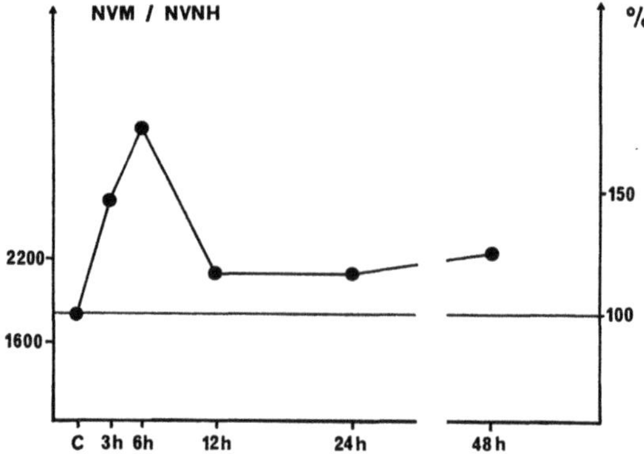

Fig. 8a. Number of mitochondria per rat hepatocyte (NVM/NVNH) after a single injection of cycloheximide. *C* Control rats

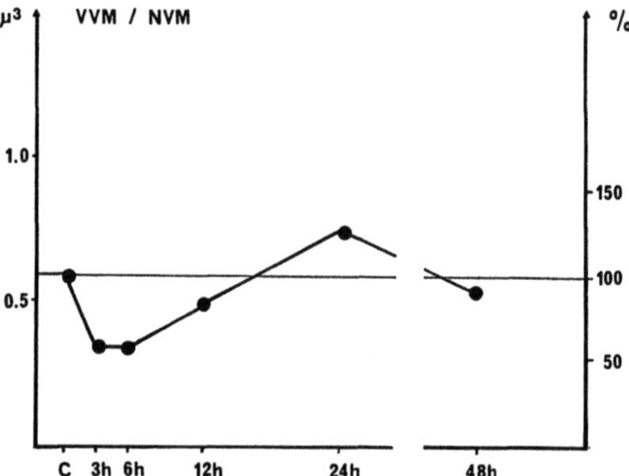

Fig. 8b. Mitochondrial single volume of rat hepatocyte (VVM/NVM) after a single injection of cycloheximide. *C* Control rats

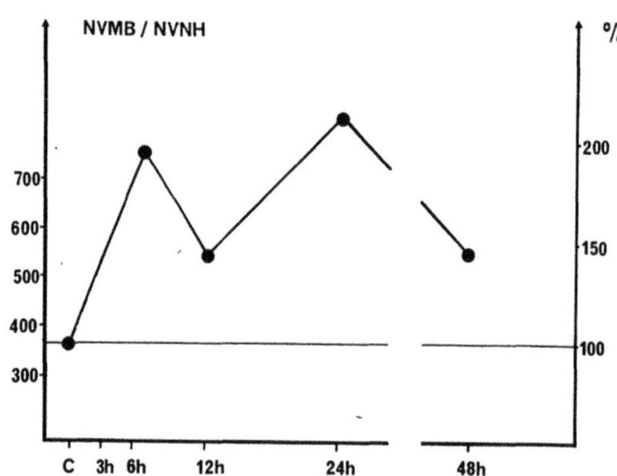

Fig. 8c. Number of microbodies per rat hepatocyte (NVMB/NVNH) after a single injection of cycloheximide. *C* Control rats

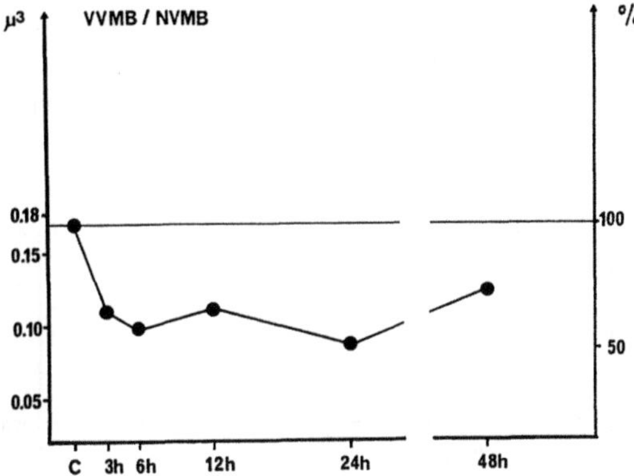

Fig. 8d. Microbody single volume of rat hepatocyte (VVMB/NVMB) after a single injection of cycloheximide. *C* Control rats

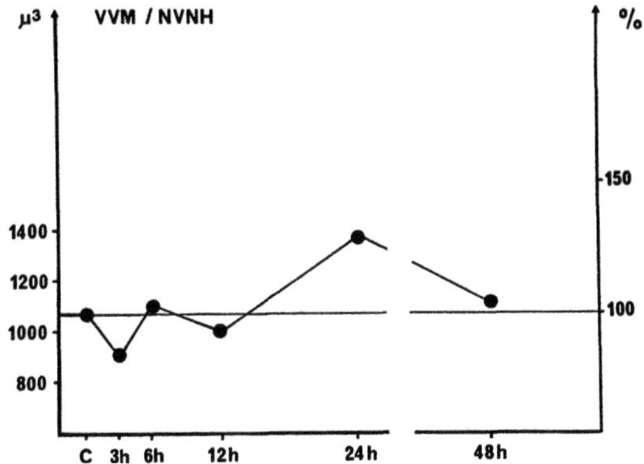

Fig. 8e. Absolute volume of mitochondria per rat hepatocyte (VVM/NVNH) after a single
injection of cycloheximide. *C* Control rats

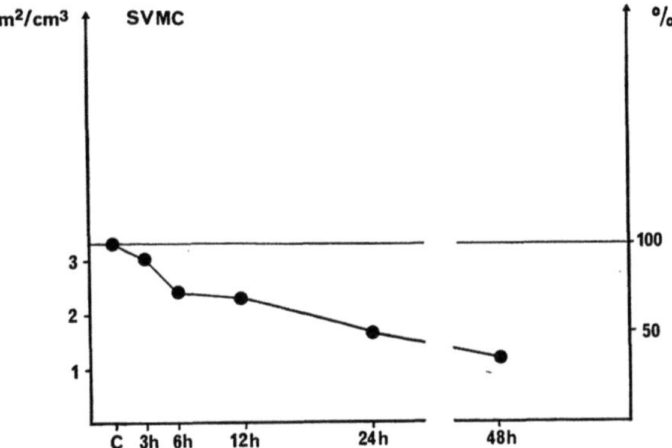

Fig. 8f. Surface density of rat mitochondrial cristae (SVMC) after a single injection of
cycloheximide. *C* Control rats

of mitochondrial proteins, preceding the division, would be inhibited (ref. Swift and Wolstenholme, 1969). Such an interpretation fits in well with the assumption that mitosis is followed by mitochondrial division (Rohr *et al.*, 1971).

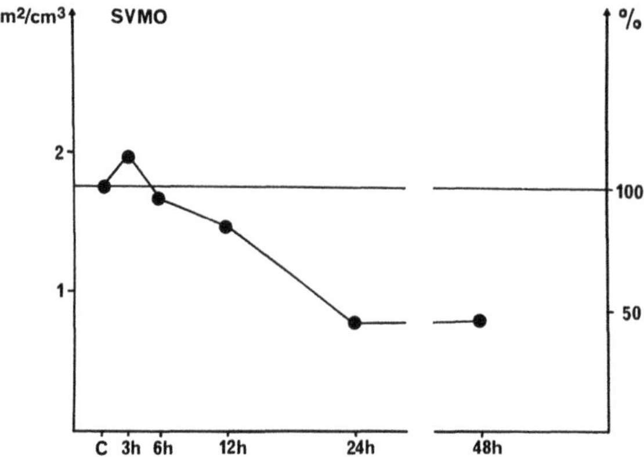

Fig. 8g. Surface density of rat mitochondrial outer membrane (SVMO) after a single injection of cycloheximide. *C* Control rats

4. The Megamitochondrion

It is known that the enzymes of the respiratory chain and the enzymes involved in oxidative phosphorylation are structurally linked with the mitochondrial inner membrane. Enzymes involved in fatty acid oxidation and protein synthesis as well as most enzymes of the citric acid cycle are encountered in the mitochondrial matrix (Borst, 1969). Therefore, the ratio of the volume of the mitochondrial matrix to the surface of the mitochondrial cristae reflects the functional state of the cell. Accordingly, mitochondria of the matrix type (of mainly metabolic function) are to be clearly distinguished from mitochondria of the cristae type (of prevailing energy generation).

The observation of sporadic giant mitochondria does not give much of an idea of their function, whereas enlarged mean single volumes of mitochondria constitute a valuable parameter which can be correlated with biochemical findings. On the basis of morphometric studies the enlargement of the single volume of mitochondria can be subdivided in the following groups:

1. Normal mitochondrial single volume: 0.70 μm^3.
2. Enlarged mitochondrial single volume: 1.5–2.0 μm^3.
3. Megamitochondrion: 2.5 μm^3.

Even under physiological conditions, different mitochondrial single volumes, according to animal species, can be observed (Riede *et al.*, 1972) (Table 1). Desert rats (Meriones crassus) normally do not take water and therefore depend on intracellular generation of oxidation water (Petter, 1951). The mitochondrial volume density of these animals is equally large as that of Wistar

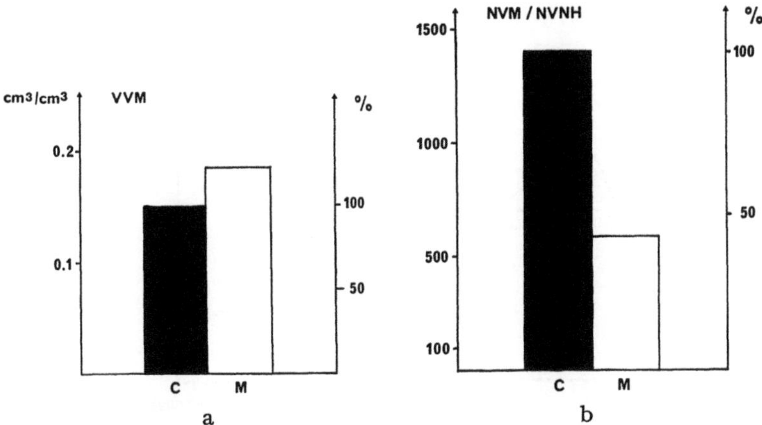

Fig. 9a. Morphometric comparison between hepatocytes of desert rats (meriones crassus) $= M$ and Wistar rats (rattus norvegicus) $= C$. Volume density of mitochondria (VVM)

Fig. 9b. Morphometric comparison between hepatocytes of desert rats (meriones crassus) $= M$ and Wistar rats (rattus norvegicus) $= C$. Number of mitochondria per hepatocyte (NVM/NVNH)

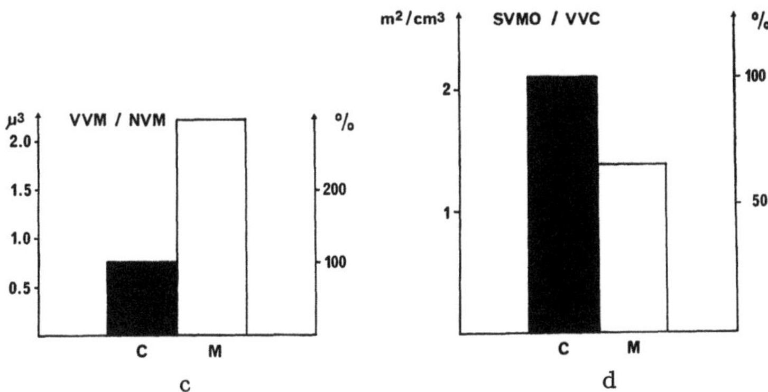

Fig. 9c. Morphometric comparison between hepatocytes of desert rats (meriones crassus) $= M$ and Wistar rats (rattus norvegicus) $= C$. Mitochondrial single volume (VVM/NVM)

Fig. 9d. Morphometric comparison between hepatocytes of desert rats (meriones crassus) $= M$ and Wistar rats (rattus norvegicus) $= C$. Surface of mitochondrial outer membrane per unit volume cytoplasm (SVMO/VVC)

rats (Fig. 9a). The chondrioma of the desert rats, however, is made up of a smaller number of larger mitochondria (Fig. 9b and c) and shows a correspondingly smaller surface of the mitochondrial outer membrane (Fig. 9d).

Under numerous experimental conditions, enlarged mitochondrial single volumes can also be shown morphometrically:

1. Riboflavin deficiency (ROHR *et al.*, 1973)
2. Tocopherol deficiency (RIEDE *et al.*, 1971, 1972)
3. Iron deficiency (GOODMAN and DALLMAN, 1971)
4. Cortisone administration (KIMBERG *et al.*, 1969)

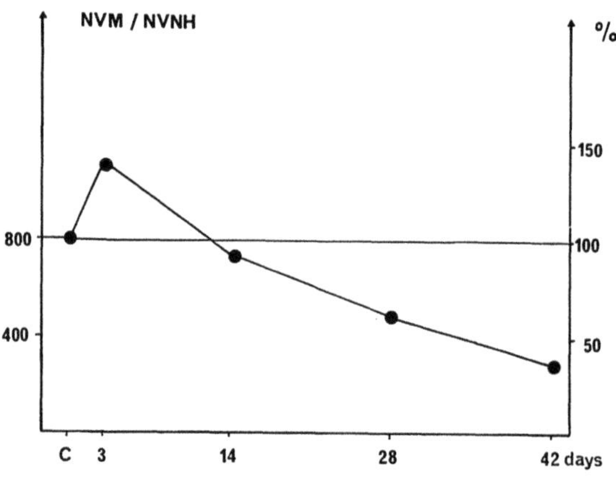

Fig. 10a. Number of mitochondria per mouse hepatocyte (NVM/NVNH) during ribo-flavin-deficiency. *C* Control mice

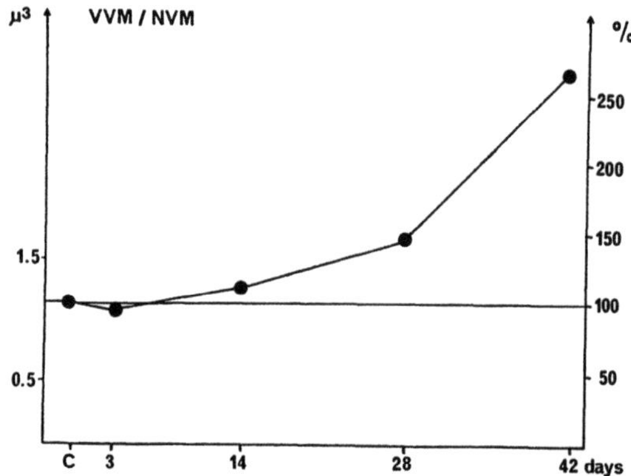

Fig. 10b. Mitochondrial single volume (VVM/NVM) of mouse hepatocyte during ribo-flavin-deficiency. *C* Control mice

5. Experimental uremia (Heitz *et al.*, 1971)
6. Administration of diet rich in orotic acid (Riede *et al.*, 1971)
7. Early phase of starvation and chronic partial starvation (Rohr *et al.*, 1973; Riede *et al.*, 1973)
8. Alcohol intoxication (Rohr *et al.*, 1971)
9. Adenine intoxication (Riede *et al.*, 1971)
10. Folic acid administration (Riede *et al.*, 1972).
11. Vitamin D deficiency (Riede *et al.*, 1973).

The reaction pattern of hepatocytes during chronic deficiency of ribo-flavin (Table 1), shown morphometrically, is biphasic. In the early phase (3–10 days) a numerical increase of mitochondria and microbodies can be observed (Fig. 10a and d).

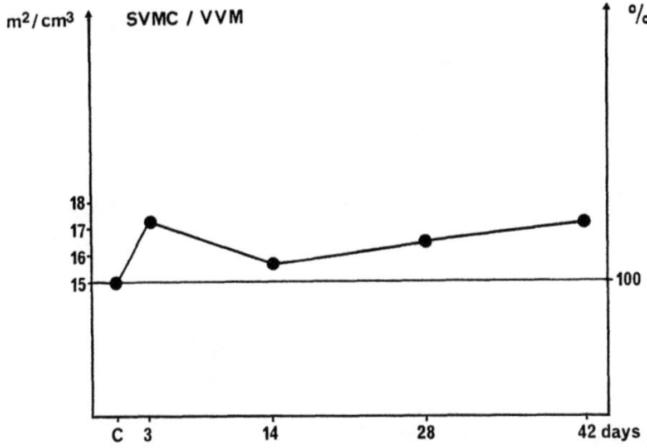

Fig. 10c. Cristae surface per unit volume mitochondrion of mouse hepatocyte (SVMC/VVM) during riboflavin-deficiency. *C* Control mice

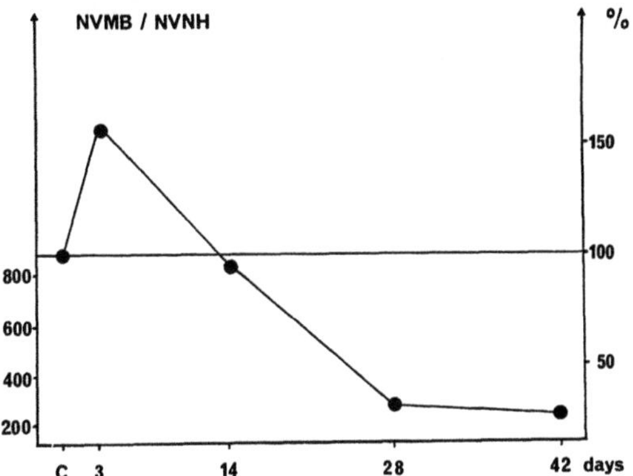

Fig. 10d. Number of microbodies per mouse hepatocyte (NVMB/NVNH) during ribo-flavin-deficiency. *C* Control mice

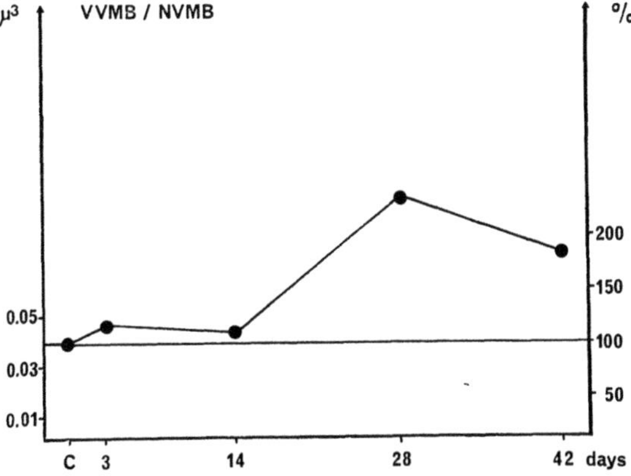

Fig. 10e. Microbody single volume of mouse hepatocyte (VVMB/NVMB) during ribo-flavin-deficiency. *C* Control mice

In the late phase (from week 4), the mean mitochondrial single volume is drastically increased (Fig. 10b). Besides, numerous giant mitochondria are found. For the pathogenesis of this mitochondrial enlargement the following processes have to be discussed (Fig. 11):

1. Inhibition of mitochondrial division. The discussion about the pathogenesis of megamitochondria induced by deficiency of riboflavin — a component of many intramitochondrial dehydrogenases — is rendered complicated

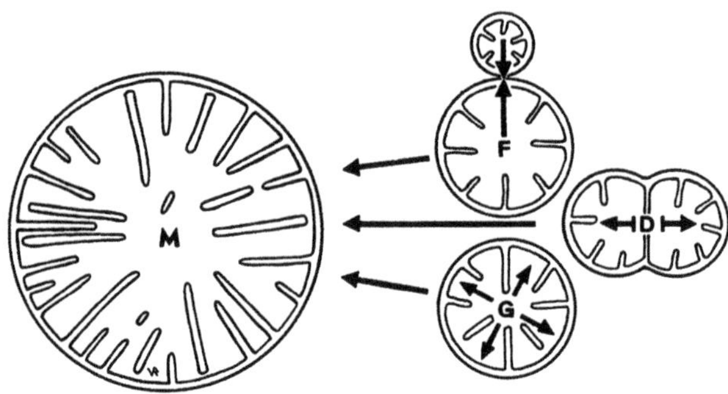

Fig. 11. Diagrammatic representation of morphogenesis of megamitochondria (M). *F* Mitochondrial fusion; *D* disturbed mitochondrial division; *G* abnormal mitochondrial growth

by the fact that at least two mitochondrial populations occur: one of a normal life-time and the other of a prolonged life-time and disturbed division activity. This is underlined by the following facts:

— Although the half-life of mitochondria amounts to about 10 days (Scarpelli *et al.*, 1971), until day 42 of administration of the diet deficient in riboflavin the mean mitochondrial single volume increases constantly.
— In the late phase, in addition to megamitochondria, numerous mitochondria of normal size can be observed.

2. Mitochondrial fusion. Such a process is conceivable, but improbable, insofar as strikingly high mitochondrial division figures occur after injection of riboflavin (Tandler *et al.*, 1969).

3. Mitochondrial swelling. This pathogenesis (Fig. 19) can definitely be excluded due to the following observations:

— Despite riboflavin deficiency, the mitochondrial matrix is up to standard.
— The cristae surface per unit volume mitochondrion remains constant during the whole experiment (Fig. 10c).

4. Abnormal mitochondrial growth. Since riboflavin deficiency is an extreme stress on the cellular metabolism, passive pathogenetic mechanisms such as inhibited division and fusion of mitochondria are more probable than overshooting mitochondrial growth.

After a nine-month diet deficient in vitamin E (Table 1) the mean single volume of mitochondria (Fig. 12b) as well as their volume density per hepatocyte are considerably increased as compared with controls (Riede *et al.*, 1972).

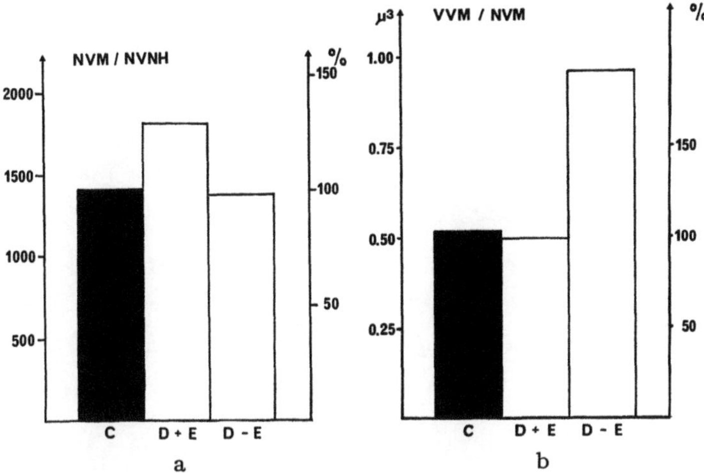

Fig. 12a. Number of mitochondria per rat hepatocyte (NVM/NVNH) during vitamin E-deficiency. *C* Control rats, *D + E* rats fed with a diet rich in carbohydrates and vitamin E added. *D–E* rats fed with a diet deficient in vitamin E

Fig. 12b. Mitochondrial single volume of rat hepatocyte (VVM/NVM) during vitamin E-deficiency. *C* Control rats, *D + E* rats fed with a diet rich in carbohydrates and vitamin E added. *D–E* rats fed with a diet deficient in vitamin E

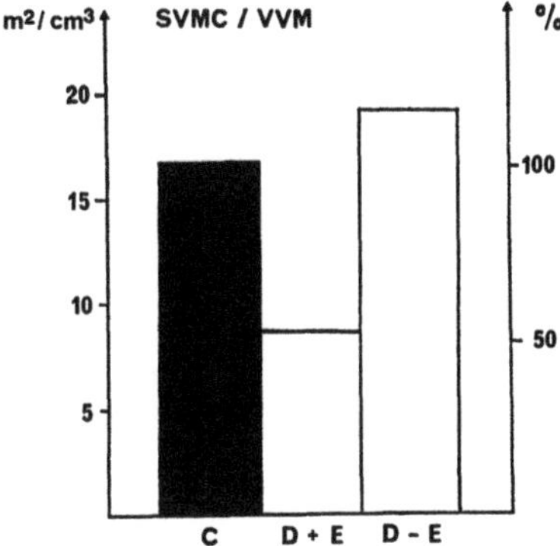

Fig. 12c. Cristae surface per unit volume mitochondrion of rat hepatocyte (SVMC/VVM) during vitaminE-deficiency. *C* Control rats, *D + E* rats fed with a diet rich in carbohydrates and vitamin E added. *D–E* rats fed with a diet deficient in vitamin E

However, the number of mitochondria per hepatocyte remains unchanged (Fig. 12a). The cristae surface per unit volume cytoplasm is also increased, but that per unit volume mitochondrion remains constant (Figs. 12c and 22).

A volume increase of the chondrioma in the case of an enlarged mitochondrial single volume can be explained by the following mechanisms (Fig. 11):

1. Retarded mitochondrial turnover. It is conceivable that single mitochondria grow due to a reduction of the mitochondrial division rate and

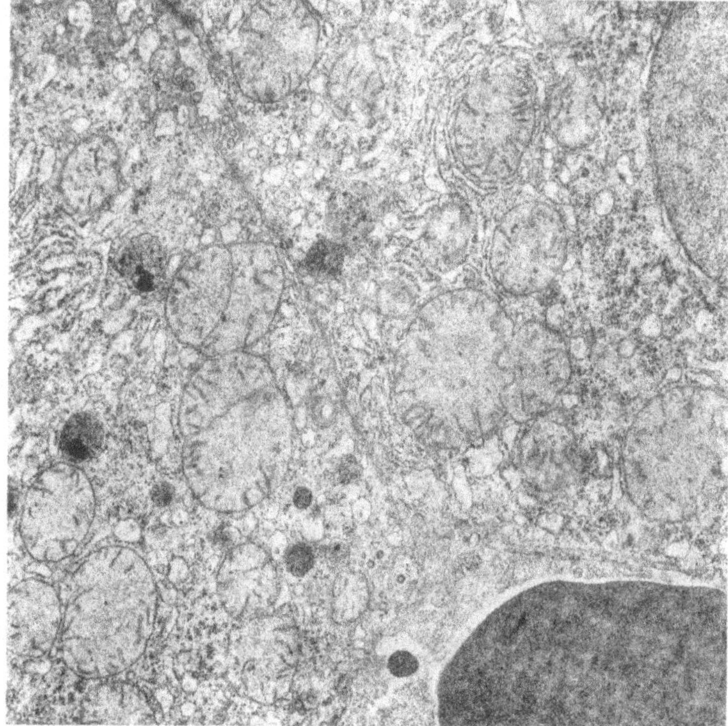

Fig. 13. Rat hepatocyte in vitamin E-deficiency. Note the herniations of mitochondrial outer-membranes in the neighboring mitochondrion 12000 ×

retarded mitochondrial break-down, so that the chondrioma is enlarged volumetrically, but not numerically.

2. Intensified mitochondrial division parallel to mitochondrial fusion. The mitochondrial division figures, frequently observed in this experiment, as well as the herniations of mitochondrial outer membranes (Fig. 13), typical of fusion processes (TANDLER *et al.*, 1968; SULKIN and SULKIN, 1962; DJACZENCO *et al.*, 1969), indicate such a mechanism. In line with the intensified mitochondrial division activity, in addition to megamitochondria, smaller mitochondria ought to be observed. However, practically the whole chondrioma in the case of vitamin E deficiency consists of enlarged mitochondria.

3. Mitochondrial swelling. Such a mechanism (Fig. 19) is unlikely for the regular electron density of the mitochondrial matrix, on the one hand, and the unchanged cristae surface density per unit volume mitochondrion, on the other (Fig. 12c). Thus, the present findings differ from those of other authors who describe mitochondrial swelling due to vitamin-E-deficiency (SULKIN and SULKIN, 1962; DJACZENCO *et al.*, 1969).

The liver parenchymal cell after administration of orotic acid (Table 1) is another example showing the enlargement of the mitochondrial single volume (RIEDE *et al.*, 1971).

Application of a diet rich in orotic acid results in a fatty liver visible even to the naked eye (NOVIKOFF *et al.*, 1966). If the reaction of the liver parenchymal cell is analysed morphometrically with regard to the disturbed metabolism, changes in the rough endoplasmic reticulum, the mitochondria, as well as the microbodies can be noticed in the course of the experiment. Under the influence of a diet rich in orotic acid the mitochondrial single volume increases, while the number of mitochondria per hepatocyte decreases (Fig. 14a and b). For the morphogenesis of this enlargement of mitochondria the following mechanisms have to be considered (Fig. 11):

1. Inhibition of mitochondrial division parallel to unimpeded synthesis and break-down of mitochondria. This pathogenetic mechanism with a reduced ATP production could be due to a purine nucleotide deficiency induced by orotic acid (WINDMUELLER, 1964; ROHEIM *et al.*, 1966). A disturbed mitochondrial function has to be assumed with regard to the decreased ATP level and the significantly reduced cytochrome oxidase activity in the liver after 7 days of feeding a diet rich in orotic acid (MARKSTEIN, 1971, personal communication). Lysosomal activity, an energy-requiring process (ARSTILA and TRUMP, 1968; ROHR *et al.*, 1970), is found to be lowered, probably as a consequence of altered mitochondrial function.

2. Mitochondrial fusion. In such a process, fusion forms and giant mitochondria are described (SUZUKI and KIKKAWA, 1969). Features of this kind are lacking in this experiment.

3. Mitochondrial swelling. This occurs due to a shift of the intra- and extramitochondrial ionic equilibrium, induced by deficiency of energy-rich substrates (WILSON and LEDUC, 1963). ATP deficiency is a constant finding after feeding a diet rich in orotic acid (WINDMUELLER, 1964). A swelling process could manifest itself in a reduced electron density of mitochondrial matrix (Fig. 19) which, however, is not observed after orotic acid administration; it is even increased (NOVIKOFF *et al.*, 1966). Furthermore, regarding the increased mitochondrial single volume, the hypothesis of such a swelling process could be favored. However, the reduction of the number of mitochondria per liver cell and the unchanged values of the cristae surface per unit volume mitochondrion ask for another causative mechanism.

An enlargement of the mitochondrial single volume can also occur in short-term experiments.

12 hours after a single injection of folic acid (Table 1) (RIEDE *et al.*, 1972), the mitochondrial single volume doubles (Fig. 15b and c). Correspondingly, the absolute volume of mitochondria per hepatocyte (Fig. 15a) increases (RIEDE *et al.*, 1972). Also in this experiment, the following pathogenetic mechanisms regarding the enlargement of the mitochondrial single volume have to be discussed (Fig. 11):

1. Mitochondrial fusion. As a rule, mitochondrial fusion occurs whenever the adhesiveness of the mitochondrial envelope becomes stronger (SUZUKI and KIKKAWA, 1969). Since after folic acid administration myelin-like structures of the mitochondrial outer membrane are observed, a change in its physico-chemical properties, and consequently also a fusion process can be assumed.

2. Mitochondrial swelling. Because of the normal electron density of the mitochondrial matrix and mainly because of the enlarged cristae surface per

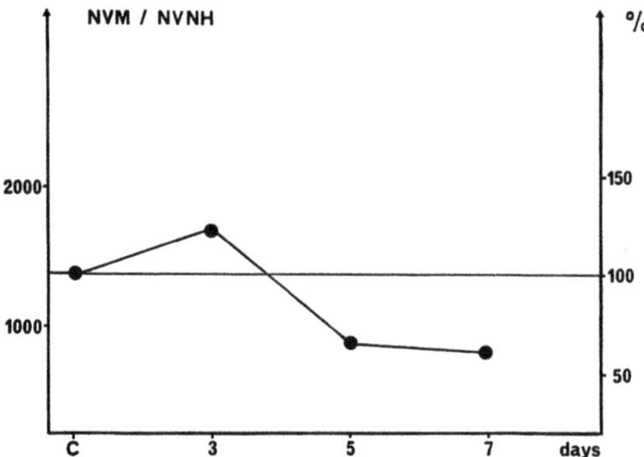

Fig. 14a. Number of mitochondria per rat hepatocyte (NVM/NVNH) after orotic acid administration. *C* Control rats

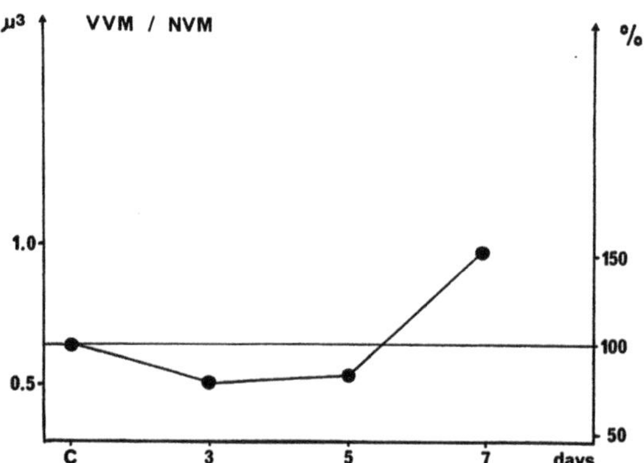

Fig. 14b. Mitochondrial single volume of rat hepatocyte (VVM/NVM) after orotic acid administration. *C* Control rats

unit volume mitochondrion (Fig. 15d), mitochondrial swelling is improbable (Fig. 19).

3. Inhibited division. Such a process does not take place due to the fact that the mitochondrial half-life amounts to about 10 days, and doubling of the mitochondrial single volume occurs only 12 hours after the injection of folic acid (Fig. 15b).

4. Accelerated growth of mitochondria. This pathogenetic mechanism seems obvious in the first analysis, since, as an enzymatic component, folic acid is involved in various anabolic processes. However, in view of the fact that the ergastoplasm shows severe changes (RIEDE *et al.*, 1972), increased synthesis of mitochondrial substance can be excluded.

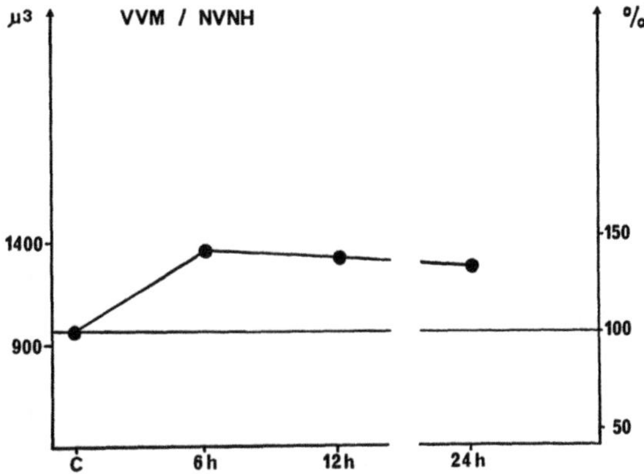

Fig. 15a. Absolute volume of mitochondria per rat hepatocyte (VVM/NVNH) after a single injection of folic acid. *C* Control rats

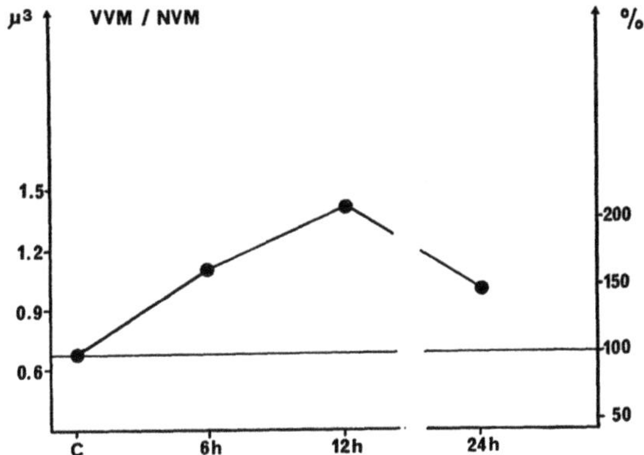

Fig. 15b. Mitochondrial single volume of rat hepatocyte (VVM/NVM) after a single injection of folic acid. *C* Control rats

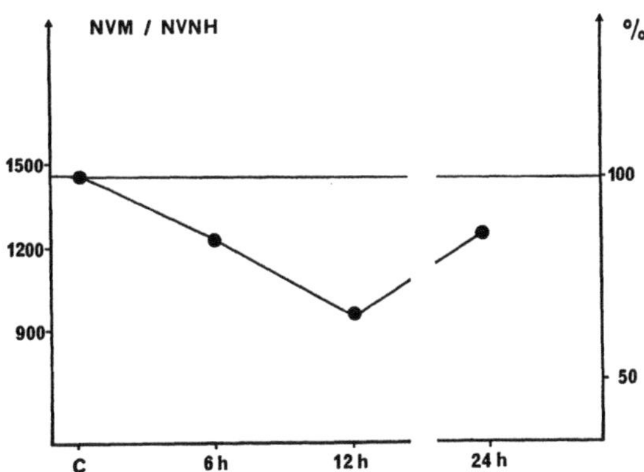

Fig. 15c. Number of mitochondria per rat hepatocyte (NVM/NVNH) after a single injection of folic acid. *C* Control rats

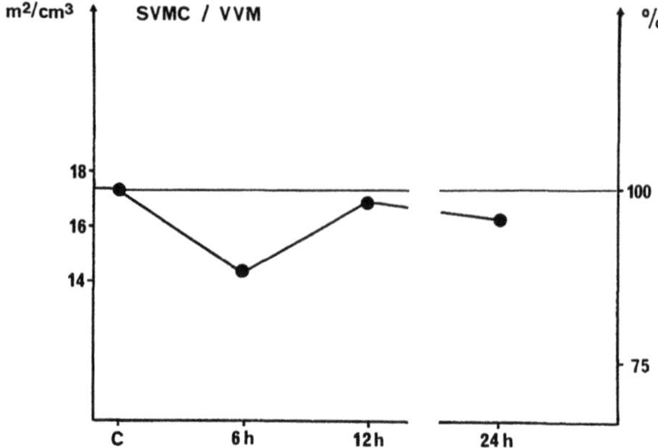

Fig. 15d. Cristae surface per unit volume mitochondrion of rat hepatocyte (SVMC/VVM) after a single injection of folic acid. *C* Control rats

5. Surface Reduction of Mitochondrial Membranes

Morphometric analyses indicate that the biogenesis of mitochondrial membranes is controlled by a mitochondrial and ribosomal protein synthesis. Cycloheximide inhibits the ribosomal protein synthesis and, consequently, also the synthesis of the mitochondrial outer membrane. The inhibiting effect of cycloheximide on the incorporation of labeled leucine into the proteins of the inner membrane may be neglected, as compared with the effect on the synthesis of the outer membrane proteins (Scarpelli *et al.*, 1971). As a matter of fact, 24 and 48 hours respectively after a single injection of cycloheximide, the surface density of the mitochondrial outer membrane decreases by 50 % (Riede *et al.*, 1971) (Fig. 8g). Therefore there is the temptation to speculate that the half-life of the mitochondrial outer membrane amounts to approximately 48 hours.

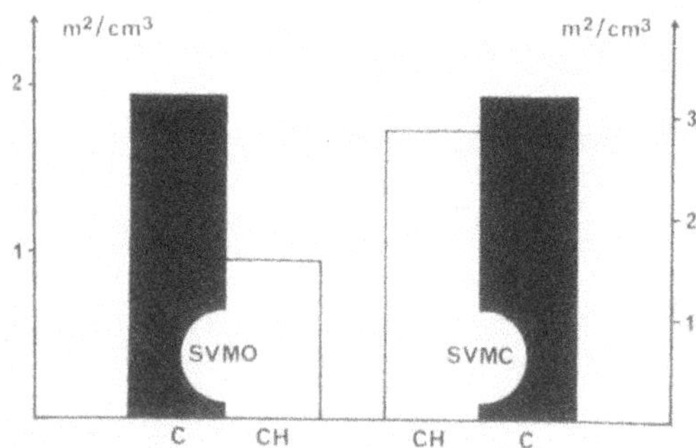

Fig. 16. Surface density of mitochondrial cristae (SVMC) and surface density of mitochondrial outer membrane (SVMO) of rat hepatocyte after 5 days of chloromycetine application. *C* Control rats

In contrast to cycloheximide, chloramphenicol inhibits not only ribosomal but also mitochondrial protein synthesis (CLARKWALKER and LINNANE, 1967) and, consequently, the formation of the mitochondrial cristae. The question of how chloramphenicol interferes in mitochondrial protein synthesis has not been clarified completely. It is assumed that chloramphenicol inhibits NADH-oxidation in the mitochondria so that ATP-production, RNA synthesis and finally also the ribosomal protein synthesis are reduced (FREEMAN and HALDAR, 1968). In any case, chloramphenicol inhibits the neogenesis of the outer and mainly inner membrane (Table 1) (COGGI and SCARPELLI, 1970). This effect can be shown morphometrically (Fig. 16).

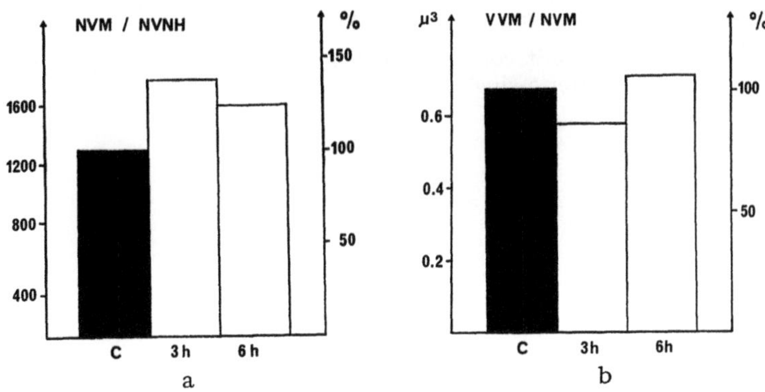

Fig. 17a. Number of mitochondria per rat hepatocyte (NVM/NVNH) after a single injection of chloromycetine. *C* Control rats

Fig. 17b. Mitochondrial single volume of rat liver (VVM/NVM) after a single injection of chloromycetine. *C* Control rats

Similar to the reaction after a single injection of cycloheximide, a few hours after the application of chloramphenicol (Table 1), the number of mitochondria per hepatocyte increases by 35–40 % of controls (Fig. 17a), whereas the mitochondrial single volume decreases (Fig. 17b). Analogous to the changes after cycloheximide, also in this case a so-called incomplete mitochondrial proliferation takes place, possibly as a response to disturbed formation of mitochondrial proteins.

6. Mitochondrial Swelling

After a single administration of malonic acid (Table 1) the cristae surface per unit volume mitochondrion is reduced (Fig. 18), and the mitochondrial matrix appears translucent in the electron microscope. Correspondingly, mito-chondrial swelling including cristolysis and matricolysis occurs (Fig. 19). This morphometric behaviour of mitochondria can be explained by the influence of exogenously applied malonic acid on the cellular metabolism. Malonic acid competitively impedes the intramitochondrial succinate dehydrogenase. Des-pite the inhibition of the oxidative metabolism by malonic acid, the surface

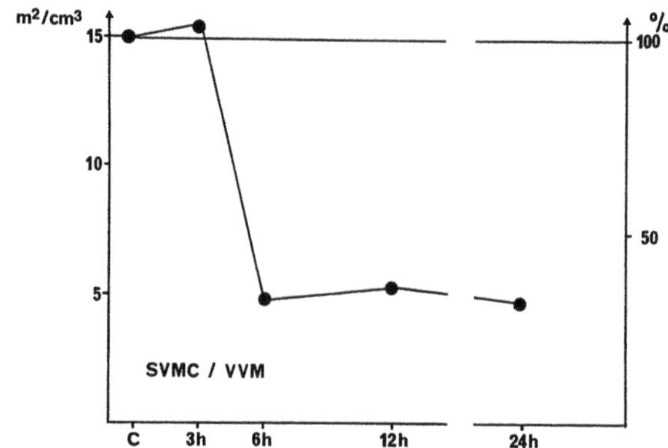

Fig. 18. Cristae surface per unit volume mitochondrion of rat hepatocyte (SVMC/VVM) after a single injection of malonic acid

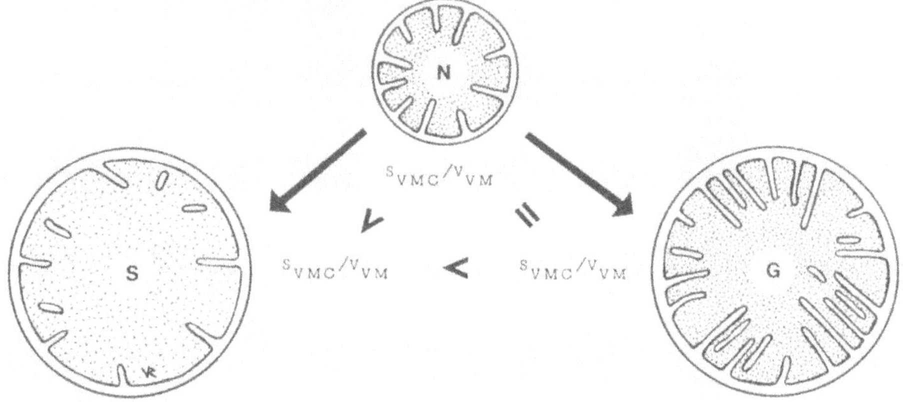

Fig. 19. Diagrammatic representation of the morphometric differentiation between mitochondrial growth (G) (with increasing quotient SVMC/VVM) and mitochondrial swelling (S) (with decreasing quotient SVMC/VVM) of normal mitochondrion (N)

ratio of mitochondrial outer membrane to mitochondrial cristae remains constant. This fact obviously shows that, notwithstanding cell injury, the point of no return has not yet been reached (Trump and Ginn, 1969), although the hepatocellular chondrioma is undergoing a decompensation phase.

A similar reaction pattern can be observed during absolute starvation (Table 1). However, in that case, the morphometric parameters of mitochondria are biphasic. The mitochondrial single volume doubles by the sixth day and increases sixfold by the ninth day (Fig. 7b). The mitochondrial number per hepatocyte remains more or less constant until the sixth day of starvation and drops drastically to 25 % of controls by the ninth day (Fig. 7a). The cristae surface per unit volume mitochondrion decreases after only 3 days of starvation but does not change considerably until the ninth day. These morphometric findings show that the chondrioma is capable of maintaining its structural integrity almost completely even during a rather long period of

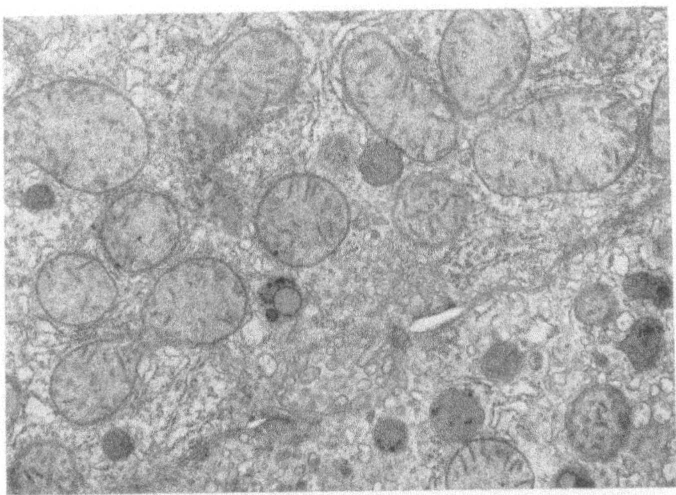

Fig. 20a. Liver mitochondria after 3 days of starvation. Note the increased mitochondrial single volume and the regular mitochondrial matrix. 10000 ×

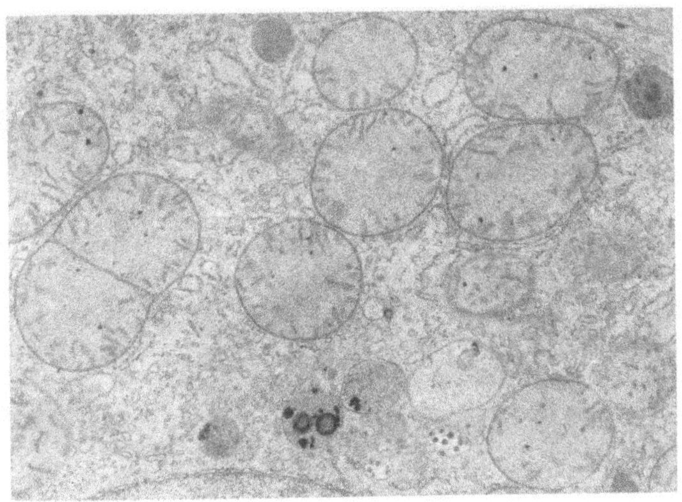

Fig. 20b. Liver mitochondria after 6 days of starvation. Note the increased mitochondrial single volume and the translucent mitochondrial matrix. 10000 ×

starvation (Fig. 20). Only after very long starvation is this compensation phase substituted by a decompensation phase, which is reflected in mitochondrial swelling, including cristolysis and matricolysis.

A similar behaviour of mitochondrial cristae can also be observed after administration of a diet rich in orotic acid (Table 1). In this case, the cristae surface per unit volume mitochondrion has doubled after 5 days of experiment and is reduced again after 7 days (RIEDE et al., 1971). Also in this experiment it is possible to observe morphometrically an early compensation phase and a late decompensation phase due to deficiency of purine nucleotides, induced by exogenously administered orotic acid (ref. FOERSTER et al., 1968). However, the decompensated hepatocellular chondrioma can be observed only bio-chemically (ref. Riede and Rohr, 1971) and not morphologically, since the mitochondrial matrix is not translucent due to matricolysis but has a higher electron density.

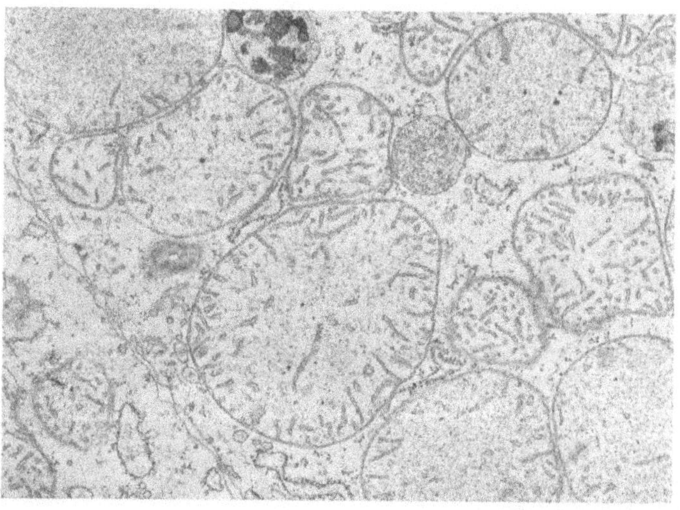

Fig. 20c. Liver mitochondria after 9 days of starvation. At this time mitochondria are extremly swollen. 10000 ×

An isolated matricolysis can be observed at least in one part of the chondrioma after a single injection of clofibrate (CPIB). As a consequence, the cristae surface per unit volume mitochondrion of Wistar rats does not show any significant change during the 12-hour experiment. In the case of desert rats, however, mitochondrial swelling with cristolysis and matricolysis can be observed, using the same experimental design (Riede et al., 1972).

7. Cristae Proliferation

The counterpart of cristolysis with a decreasing quotient SVMC/VVM is the enlargement of the cristae surface, a process in which the quotient SVMC/VVM increases (Fig. 19). An enlargement of the cristae surface is characteristic of the adaptation phase after a functional overload.

D-penicillamine is a chelating agent almost specific for copper, binding the metal present in the body and inhibiting the intestinal uptake. The human body normally contains about 100 mg of copper, 90 % of which is bound to ceruloplasmin. This copper-protein complex acts as a ferro-oxidase in synthesizing iron-containing enzymes in the respiratory chain. Copper is a constituent of oxidases, e.g. xanthine oxidase, uricase, D-amino acid oxidase of microbodies and cytochrome oxidase of mitochondrial cristae. All these enzymes, except D-amino acid oxidase, function as so-called terminal oxidases in the last step of biological oxidation processes (ref. Riede et al., 1971).

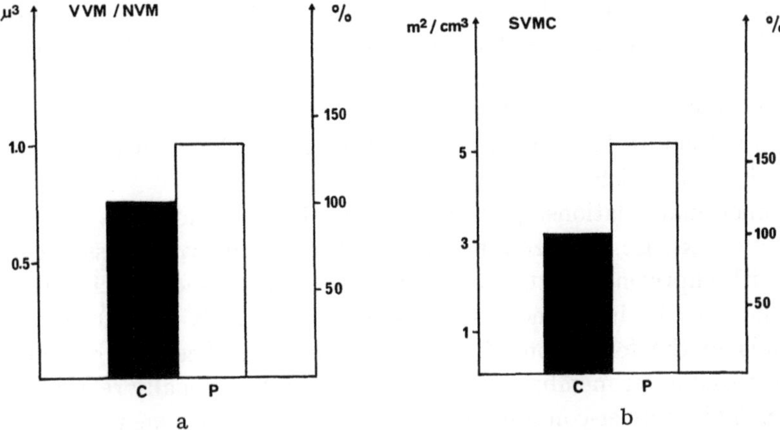

Fig. 21a. Mitochondrial single volume of rat liver (VVM/NVM) after 7 weeks of D-penicillamine administration (*P*). *C* Control rats

Fig. 21b. Surface density of mitochondrial cristae of rat liver (SVMC) after 7 weeks of D-penicillamine administration (*P*). *C* Control rats

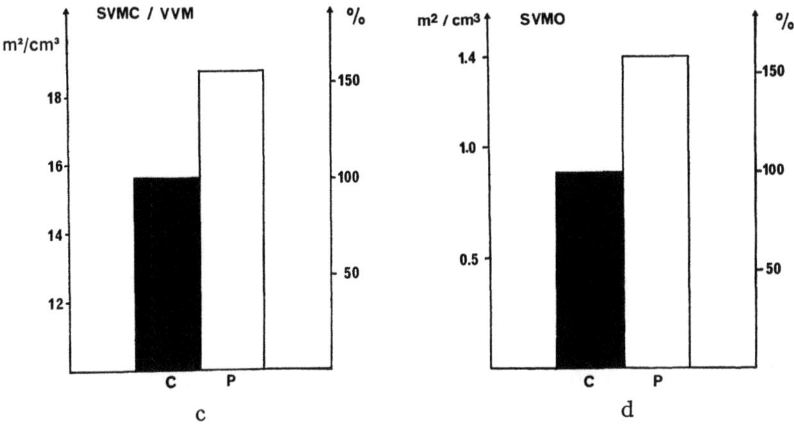

Fig. 21c. Cristae surface per unit volume mitochondrion of rat liver (SVMC/VVM) after 7 weeks of D-penicillamine administration (*P*). *C* Control rats

Fig. 21d. Surface density of mitochondrial outer membrane of rat liver (SVMO) after 7 weeks of D-penicillamine administration (*P*). *C* Control rats

In a long-term experiment (Table 1), these properties of D-penicillamine lead one to expect a corresponding reaction of the mitochondrial cristae and microbodies. As a matter of fact, after 7 weeks of D-penicillamine treatment significant morphometric changes of the copper-containing cell compartments can be observed (RIEDE *et al.*, 1971). While the mitochondrial single volume has increased only slightly, the surface-density of outer membranes and cristae is considerably higher, and the cristae surface per unit volume mitochondrion has doubled (Fig. 21a–d).

These findings show when and how hepatocytes react to copper deficiency. The critical time with regard to the turnover of structurally-bound copper, of iron, manganese and essential fatty acids is between week 5 and 8 (Dallman and Goodman, 1971; Hurley et al., 1970; Wilson and Leduc, 1963; Smithson, 1969), a fact which is proved by the striking surface enlargement of mitochondrial cristae.

A functional relationship between this alteration and the cuproenzyme cytochrome oxidase, localized in mitochondrial cristae can be assumed. Treatment with cuprizone (Suzuki and Kikkawa, 1969), another chelating agent for copper, results in an increase in cristae of normally-shaped mitochondria and leads to the formation of giant mitochondria. The enlargement of the mitochondrial outer membrane is supposed to be functionally related to amine oxidase. This copper-containing enzyme of the outer membrane may be altered by the cuprizone-induced copper deficiency (Suzuki and Kikkawa, 1969). On the other hand, a loss of mitochondrial membranes in giant mitochondria after cuprizone treatment has been reported. In our experiments with penicillamine, however, as well as after a diet deficient in copper (Goodman and Dallman, 1967), the enlargement of mitochondria was not conspicuous, and a loss of membranes could not be confirmed. These differences suggest that the 2 copper-chelating agents, penicillamine and cuprizone must have different sites of action at the subcellular level (Riede et al., 1971).

An enlargement of the cristae surface in the course of extreme stress on the metabolism can be observed morphometrically even after 9 months of administration of a diet deficient in vitamin E (Table 1). A comparison between the mitochondria of the rats deficient in vitamin E and those of the rats fed with a diet rich in carbohydrates with tocopherol added (diet controls) shows diametrical values of the cristae surfaces (Riede et al., 1972). The cristae surface per unit volume mitochondrion and also per unit volume cytoplasm doubles under the influence of vitamin-E-deficiency, whereas the corresponding values are reduced by 50 % in the case of the diet controls (Fig. 22). These morphometric changes of mitochondrial cristae suggest that vitamin-E-deficiency induces relative deficiency of essential fatty acids. The following facts underline this assumption:

1. The larger part of mitochondrial lipids consists of unsaturated fatty acids (ref. Borst, 1969).

2. Tocopherol is a structural component of mitochondria (Tappel, 1962).

3. Due to tocopherol deficiency, the antioxidative effect on the unsaturated mitochondrial fatty acids is eliminated (Tappel, 1962).

The question of which mechanism induces this kind of cristae proliferation has not been answered clearly up to now. Wilson and Leduc (1963) interpreted the mitochondrial enlargement in essential fatty acid deficiency as the consequence of a negative feed-back mechanism: The altered molecular architecture of mitochondrial membranes is presumed to be due to a replacement of the lacking essential fatty acids by saturated ones. As a result, the oxidative phosphorylation, and consequently the production of ATP, would be diminished. Thus, the main source of cell energy would be exhausted. This lack of energy would then act as a trigger for the growth of additional mitochondrial cristae.

It has been suggested that the surface area of mitochondrial membranes in relation to that of the limiting cell membrane is indicative of the respiration rate characteristic of the cell (LEHNINGER, 1964). Accordingly, if this

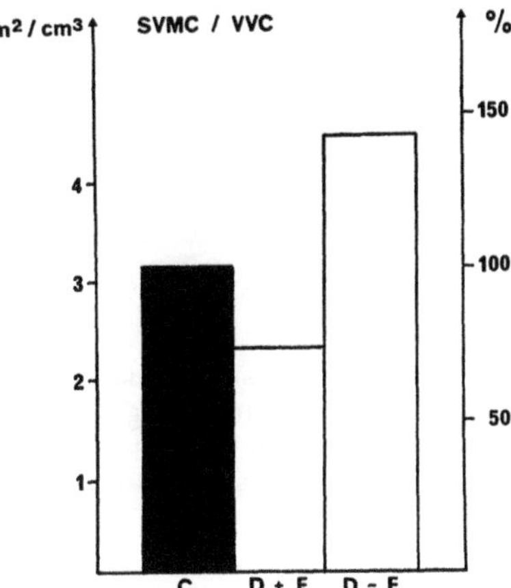

Fig. 22. Cristae surface per unit volume cytoplasm of rat hepatocytes after SVMC/VVC Vitamin E-deficiency. *C* Control rats; *D + E* Rat fed with a diet rich in carbohydrates and vitamin E added; *D–E* rats fed with a diet rich in carbohydrates and deficient in vitamin E

ratio is high, respiration is also high. With regard to the hepatocyte, this quotient is estimated morphometrically by the cristae surface per unit volume cytoplasm. Since the surface density of mitochondrial cristae is drastically increased in the case of vitamin-E deficiency and after penicillamine administration, cell respiration would also have to be intensified. However, as a matter of fact, the P:O quotient decreases in the case of vitamin-E-deficiency (TAPPEL, 1962). For these reasons, it can be concluded that the cristae proliferation observed morphometrically must be interpreted as defective compensation of the disturbed oxidative metabolism, either by inefficient, membrane-bound enzymes or by structurally altered membranes.

Similar mitochondrial cristael changes ar found in Vitamin D-deficiency (RIEDE *et al.*, 1973).

VI. Morphometric Transformation of the Hepatic Chondrioma

An analysis of the morphometric changes in relation to time allows to draw up the following reaction scheme of the hepatocellular chondrioma (Fig. 23):

In the early phase of an experiment, in many cases an increase of the mitochondrial number per hepatocyte accompanied by a diminishing mito-

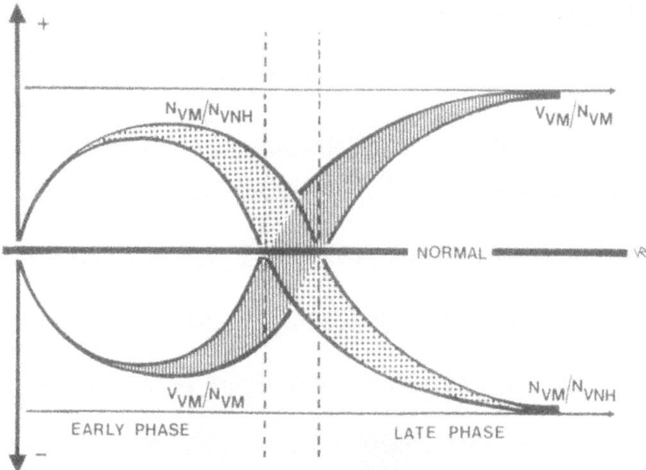

Fig. 23. Morphometric transformation of hepatocellular chondrioma (VVM/NVNH). In the early phase of a cell reaction mitochondrial single volume (VVM/NVM) decreases and increases in the late phase. The number of mitochondria per hepatocyte (NVM/NVNH) shows a diametrical pattern

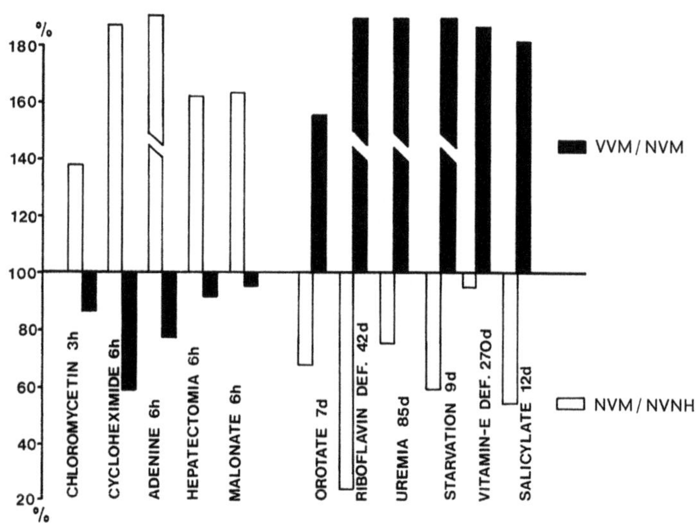

Fig. 24. Diagrammatic representation of the correlation of the mitochondrial single volume (VVM/NVM) and the mitochondrial number per hepatocyte (NVM/NVNH) in short-term and long-term experiments (as percent of the controls)

chondrial single volume can be observed. However, the volume density of mitochondria usually remains constant. In the late phase of an experiment, these morphometric parameters show diametrical values: The mitochondrial single volume increases, while the mean mitochondrial number per hepatocyte decreases (Fig. 24).

This stereotype reaction pattern of mitochondria is based on a morphometric transformation of the chondrioma. In the early phase, the increase of the mitochondrial number is the most important change. This process is the consequence of incomplete proliferation. In the late phase, the increase of the mitochondrial single volume is the most striking feature.

The question of the functional significance of the transformation the chondrioma undergoes in the early phase of cell reaction requires further clarification. It is conceivable that the surface of the mitochondrial outer membrane, important for the transmitochondrial passage, is enlarged by this transformation, a process which could be explained by the fact that the surface of a high number of small spheres is larger than that of a small number of large spheres.

Usually, the transformation of the chondrioma in the late phase of cell reaction is observed as an extreme state. It seems to be a stage of tolerance at which the chondrioma is capable of maintaining a cellular "vita minima". In this connection, the cristae surface per unit volume mitochondrion plays a decisive role. Since the single mitochondrion is a functional unit, in a transformation where mitochondrial single volumes are enlarged, the interaction of the various metabolic processes in mitochondria is possibly optimized. However, in the course of cell injury such a chondrioma seems to get near the point of no return (TRUMP and GINN, 1969). An example is the chondrioma of desert rats (RIEDE et al., 1971), which consists of a smaller number of larger mitochondria than in Wistar rats. Whereas the cristae surface per unit volume mitochondrion of Wistar rats hardly changes after a single CPIB injection, in desert rats cristolysis occurs after a few hours (RIEDE et al., 1972).

VII. Morphometric Correlations between Mitochondria and Microbodies

Analogous to the chondrioma, the aggregate of microbodies per hepatocyte might be called "peroxysoma". Accordingly, microbodies show the following morphometric changes:

1. Increase or decrease of the microbody single volume (Fig. 8 and 10)
2. Microbody proliferation (Fig. 8 and 10)
3. Morphometric transformation of the peroxysoma.

These possibilities of reaction enable microbodies to respond with a pattern similar to that of mitochondria to altered cellular metabolism. As a matter of fact, under many experimental conditions microbodies react in a similar way to mitochondria (Fig. 25). This reaction pattern, in many cases analogous to that of mitochondria, indicates a close functional relationship between microbodies and mitochondria, such as suggested in the concept of peroxysomes by DE DUVE and co-workers.

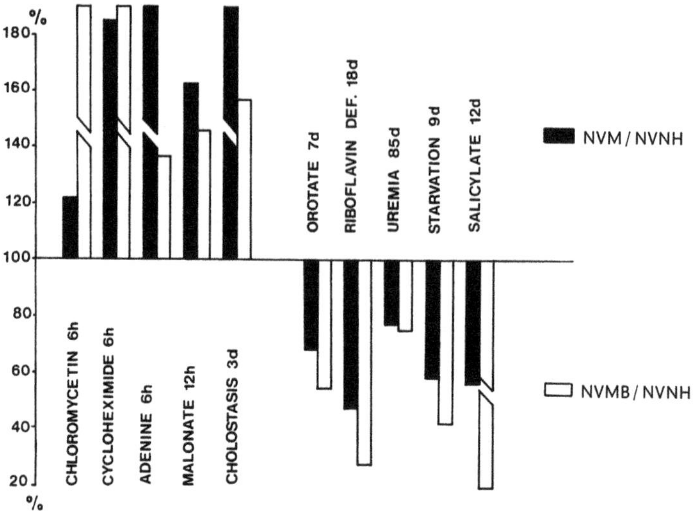

Fig. 25. Diagrammatic representation of the correlation of the mitochondrial number NVM/NVNH and microbody number per hepatocyte NVMB/NVNH in short-term and long-term experiments (as percent of the controls)

VIII. Summary and Conclusions

Under experimental conditions, liver mitochondria show the following morphometric changes:

1. Mitochondrial proliferation: increase in number
2. Megamitochondria: increase in volume
3. Cristae proliferation: increase in surface
4. Surface reduction of mitochondrial membranes.

As a rule, mitochondrial proliferation characterizes the early phase, while megamitochondria and cristae proliferation are typical of the late phase of cellular response to cell injury.

Mitochondria contain DNA and RNA. Thus, mitochondria enjoy a certain degree of autonomy within the cell. Therefore, it is possible to establish analogies between the morphometric changes of mitochondria and those of nuclei. In the adult rat liver most hepatocytes are polyploid and, therefore, show enlarged nuclear volumes which can be assigned to various categories of nuclei. The highest degree of ploidy is observed in pericentral hepatocytes. Consequently, it is conceivable that liver mitochondria are also of differing DNA-content. The existence of different mitochondrial populations, seen repeatedly in our experiments, could correspond to such assumption.

Therefore in megamitochondria the DNA-content could be increased. Another explanation of the pathogenesis of megamitochondria is the absence of a mechanism or substance which might trigger mitochondrial division. It may well be that at least some of the B vitamins act as rate-limiting factors in mitochondrial partition. Like normal cell division, mitochondrial division is preceded by DNA replication and synthesis of mitochondrial matrix and membrane proteins. All these processes of synthesis consume energy. The mitochondria resulting from mitochondrial proliferation, which is observed in the case of inhibition of the oxidative metabolism or of the mitochondrial protein synthesis, are therefore found to be incomplete structurally and functionally. Such a mitochondrial division is due to a partition process which corresponds to amitosis without preceding DNA replication. The normalization of mitochondria, e.g. during refeeding after starvation, can finally be explained by this kind of 'amitotic' partition processes of mitochondria.

References

ALTMANN, R.: Die Elementarorganismen und ihre Beziehungen zu den Zellen, S. 145. Leipzig: Veit 1890.

ARSTILA, A. U., TRUMP, B. F.: Studies on cellular autophagocytosis. The formation of autophagic vacuoles in the liver after glucagon administration. Amer. J. Path. 53, 687–734 (1968).

BECKER, F. F., LANE, B. P.: Regeneration of the mammalian liver. I. Autophagocytosis during dedifferentiation of the cell in preparation for cell division. Amer. J. Path. 47, 783–801 (1965).

BECKER, F. F., LANE, B. P.: Regeneration of the mammalian liver. VI. Retention of phenobarbital-induced cytoplasmic alterations in dividing hepatocytes. Amer. J. Path. 52, 211–221 (1968).

BERGERON, M., DROZ, B.: Protein renewal in mitochondria as revealed by electron microscopy. J. Ultrastruct. Res. 26, 17–30 (1969).

BORST, P., KROONE, A. M. RUTTENBERG G. J. C. M.: Genetic elements: properties and function (ed. D. SHUGER), p. 81–116. London and Warsaw: Academic Press, P. W. N. 1967.

CLARK-WALKER, G. D., LINNANE, A. W.: The biogenesis of mitochondria in saccharomyces cerevisiae. A comparison between cytoplasmic respiratory-deficient mutant yeast and chloramphenicol-inhibited wold type cells. J. Cell Biol. 34, 1–14 (1967).

CLERICI, E., CAMMARANO, P., MOCARELLI, P.: Protein synthesis in the early stages of liver regeneration. Experientia (Basel) 21, 143–144 (1965).

COGGI, G., SCARPELLI, D. G.: Biogenesis of mitochondrial membranes: Biochemical and morphological evidence of two protein-synthesizing systems. Proc. Soc. exp. Biol. (N.Y.) 134, 328–331 (1970).

DALLMAN, P. R., GOODMAN, J. R.: The effects of iron deficiency on the hepatocyte: a biochemical and ultrastructural study. J. Cell Biol. 48, 79–90 (1971).

DJACZENCO, W., GRABSKA, J., URBANOVICZ, M., PEZZI, R.: Peculiar mitochondrial forms in the liver parenchymal cells of rats kept on vitamin-E-deficient diet. J. Microsc. 8, 139–144 (1968).

ENNIS, H. L., LUBIN, M.: Cycloheximide. Aspects of inhibition of protein synthesis in mammalian cells. Science 146, 1474–1492 (1964).

FLETCHER, M. J., SANADI, D. R.: Turnover of rat liver mitochondria. Biochem. biophys. Acta (Amst.) 51, 356–360 (1961).

FOERSTER, E., HOLLDORF, A. M., FALK, H.: Probleme der Stoffwechselregulation in der Leber. III. Regulationsmechanismen im Lipid-Stoffwechsel. Acta hepato-splenol. (Stuttg.) 15, 291–307 (1968).

FORBUS, W. D.: Reaction to injury; pathology for students of disease. Baltimore: Williams and Wilkins Co. 1943.

Freeman, K. B., Haldar, D.: The inhibition of mammalian mitochondrial NADH oxidation by chloramphenicol and its isomers and analogues. Canad. J. Biochem. **46**, 1003–1014 (1968).

Heitz, Ph., Meier, P., Riede, U. N.: Ultrastrukturell-morphometrische Veränderungen der Leberparenchymzelle der Ratte bei experimentellem chronischem urämischem Syndrom. Path. europ. **6**, 433–444 (1971).

Higgins, G. M., Anderson, R. M.: Experimental pathology of the liver. I. Restoration of the liver of the white rat following partial surgical removal. Arch. Path. **12**, 186–202 (1931).

Hurley, L. S., Theriault, L. L., Dreosti, I. E.: Liver mitochondria from manganese-deficient and pallid mice: Function and ultrastructure. Science **170**, 1316–1318 (1970).

Kimberg, D. V., Loud, A. V., Wiener, J.: Cortisone-induced alteration in mitochondrial function and structure. J. Cell Biol. **37**, 63–79 (1968).

Kuramatsu, M., Busch, H.: Effects of thioacetamide on metabolism of proteins of normal and regenerating liver. Cancer Res. **22**, 1100–1104 (1962).

Lehninger, A. L.: A quantitative stereological description of the ultrastructure of normal rat liver parenchymal cells. J. Cell Biol. **37**, 27–46 (1968).

Madreiter, H., Mittermayer, Ch., Osieka, R.: ^{3}H-thymidine incorporation into mitochondria of synchronized mouse fibroblasts. Beitr. Path. **145**, 249–255 (1972).

Majumdar, A., Tsukada, C. K., Liebermann, I.: Liver protein synthesis after partial hepatectomy and acute stress. J. biol. Chem. **242**, 700–704 (1967).

Markstein, R.: Beiträge zur Klärung des Wirkungsmechanismus von α-Tocopherol. Inaug.-Diss. Universität Basel (1971).

Novikoff, A. B., Roheim, P. S., Quintana, N.: Changes in rat liver cells induced by orotic acid feeding. Lab. Invest. **15**, 27–49 (1966).

Petter, F.: Notes sur quelques rongeurs du Sahara occidental. Mammalia (Paris) **15**, 69–72 (1951).

Reith, A., Schueler, B., Vogell, W.: Quantitative und qualitative elektronenmikroskopische Untersuchungen zur Struktur des Leberläppchens normaler Ratten. Z. Zellforsch. **89**, 225–240 (1968).

Riede, U. N., Ettlin, Ch., Allmen, R. von, Rohr, H. P.: Vergleichende ultrastrukturell-morphometrische Untersuchungen zwischen der Leberparenchymzelle der Wistarratte (Rattus norvegicus) und der Wüstenratte (Meriones crassus) nach einer einmaligen CPIB (Clofibrat)-Verabreichung. Naunyn-Schmiedeberg's Arch. Pharmacol. **272**, 336–350 (1972).

Riede, U. N., Küpfer, A., Rasser, Y., Rupp, S., Rohr, H. P.: Vergleichende ultrastrukturell-morphometrische Untersuchungen der Leberparenchymzellen der Wistarratten (Rattus norvegicus) und der Wüstenratten (Meriones crassus). Z. Zellforsch. **123**, 240–250 (1972).

Riede, U. N., Leibundgut, U., Rohr, H. P.: Ultrastruktureller und morphometrischer Nachweis einer durch Vitamin D-Mangel induzierten Störung im oxydativen Stoffwechsel. Exp. Cell res. (1973) in press.

Riede, U. N., Markstein, R., Bianchi, L., Rohr, H. P.: Influence of vitamin-E-deficiency on rat hepatocytes. A morphometric and biochemical analyses. Proc. roy. micr. Soc. **6**, 25 (1971).

Riede, U. N., Senn, E., Rohr, H. P.: Morphometrische Untersuchung der Lebermitochondrien beim Vitamin-E-Mangel der Ratte. Cytobiologie **5**, 181–189 (1972).

Riede, U. N., Stitny, C., Althaus, S., Rohr, H. P.: Ultrastrukturell-morphometrische Untersuchungen der Rattenparenchymzelle nach chronischer Vitamin-E-Mangeldiät. Beitr. Path. **145**, 24–36 (1972).

Riede, U. N., Strässle, H., Bianchi, L., Rohr, H. P.: Ultrastructural-morphometric analysis of rat liver cell after orotic acid administration. Exp. molec. Path. **15**, 231–280 (1971).

Riede, U. N., Widmer, A. E., Bianchi, L., Molnar, J., Rohr, H. P.: Ultrastrukturell-morphometrische Untersuchungen an der Rattenleberparenchymzelle nach akuter Adenin-Intoxikation. Path. europ. **5**, 1–18 (1971).

Roheim, P. S., Switzer, S., Girard, A., Eder, H. A.: The mechanism of inhibition of lipoprotein synthesis by orotic acid. Biochem. biophys. Res. Commun. **20**, 416 (1965).

Roheim, P. S., Switzer, S., Girard, A., Eder, H. A.: Alterations of lipoprotein metabolism in orotic acid-induced fatty liver. Lab. Invest. **15**, 21–23 (1966).

ROHR, H. P., ANDERES, C., BIANCHI, L.: Ultrastrukturell-morphometrische Untersuchungen an der Leberparenchymzelle der Ratte nach Glucagon-Gabe (unter besonderer Berücksichtigung lysosomaler Funktionsformen). Beitr. Path. **141**, 313–326 (1970).

ROHR, H. P., BIANCHI, L., RIEDE U. N.: Autoradiographic-morphometric study on mitochondrial division in regenerating liver cell (abstract). Proc. roy. micr. Soc. **6**, 25 (1971).

ROHR, H. P., BIANCHI, L., STOCKMANN, F., HUNSTAD, A. C.: Morphometrische Untersuchungen über den Einfluß der physiologischen Tagesschwankung auf die Ultrastruktur der Leber. Schweiz. med. Wschr. **99**, 1163 (1969).

ROHR, H. P., HUNSTAD, A. C., BIANCHI, L., ECKERT, H.: Morphometrisch-ultrastrukturelle Untersuchungen über die durch die Tageszeit induzierten Veränderungen der Rattenleberparenchymzelle. Acta anat. (Basel) **76**, 102–111 (1970).

ROHR, H. P., STREBEL, J., BIANCHI, L.: Ultrastrukturell-morphometrische Untersuchungen an der Rattenleberparenchymzelle in der Frühphase der Regeneration nach partieller Hepatektomie. Beitr. Path. **141**, 52–74 (1970).

ROHR, H. P., WIRZ, A., HENNING, L. Ch., BIANCHI, L.: Ultrastructural and morphometric study of the perinatal rat liver cell; Septième Congr. Internat. Microsc. Electron. Grenoble, vol. III, p. 489 (1970).

ROHR, H. P., WIRZ, A., HENNING, L. Ch., RIEDE, U. N., BIANCHI, L.: Morphometric analysis of the rat liver cell in the perinatal period. Lab. Invest. **24**, 128–139 (1971).

SCARPELLI, D. G., CHIGA, M., HAYNES, E.: Experimental modification of mitochondrial biogenesis in rat liver cells. In: Cell membranes: Biological and pathological aspects (G. W. Richter and D. G. Scarpelli, eds.). Baltimore: Williams and Wilkins Co. 1971.

SMITHSON, J. E.: The effects of essential fatty acid deficiency on the liver mitochondria of rat and mouse. Lab. Invest. **20**, 207–212 (1969).

STOCKMANN, F., BIANCHI, L., ROHR, H. P., ECKERT, H.: Morphometrische Untersuchungen an der Rattenleberparenchymzelle nach Anwendung verschiedener Fixationspuffer. Experientia (Basel) **26**, 174–175 (1970).

SULKIN, M., SULKIN, D.: Mitochondrial alterations in liver cells following vitamin-E-deficiency. Fifth internat. Congr. f. Electron Microscopy, W–8 (1962).

SUZUKI, K., KIKKAWA, Y.: Status spongiosus of CNS and hepatic changes induced by cuprizone (biscyclohexamineoxalylhydrazone). Amer. J. Path. **54**, 307–326 (1969).

SWIFT, H., WOLSTENHOLME, D. R.: Mitochondria and chloroplasts: nucleic acids and the problem of biogenesis (genetics and biology). In: Handbook of molecular cytology (A Lima-de-Faria, ed.). Amsterdam–London: North-Holland Publishing Company 1969.

TANDLER, B., ERLANDSON, R. A., EYNDER, E. L.: Riboflavin and mouse hepatic cell structure and function: I. Ultrastructural alterations in simple deficiency. Amer. J. Path. **52**, 69–95 (1968).

TANDLER, B., ERLANDSON, A., SMITH, L., WYNDLER, L.: Riboflavin and mouse hepatic cell structure and function. II. Division of mitochondria during recovery from simple deficiency. J. Cell Biol. **41**, 477–493 (1969).

TAPPEL, A. L.: Vitamin E as the biological lipid antioxidant. In: R. S. HARRIS, I. G. WOOL, G. F. MARRIAN, K. THIMANN (eds.), Vitamins and hormones. Advances in research and applications, vol. 20, p. 493–509. New York–London: Academic Press 1962.

TRUMP, B. F., ARSTILA, A. U.: Cell injury and cell death. In: Pathobiology. London: Oxford Press 1971.

TRUMP, B. F., GINN, F. L.: The pathogenesis of subcellular reaction to lethal injury. In: Methods and achievements in experimental pathology, vol. IV, p. 1–29 (E. Bajusz, and G. Jasmin, eds.). Chicago: Yearbook Medical Publishers 1969.

TSUKADA, K., LIEBERMANN, I.: Protein synthesis by liver polyribosomes after partial hepatectomy. Biochem. biophys. Res. Commun. **19**, 702–707 (1965).

WEIBEL, E. R.: Stereological principles for morphometry in electron microscopic cytology. Int. Rev. Cytol. **26**, 235–302 (1969).

WEIBEL, E. R., GOMEZ, D. M.: A principle for counting tissue structures on random sections. J. appl. Physiol. **17**, 343–348 (1967).

WEIBEL, E. R., KISTLER, G. S., SCHERLE, W. F.: Practical stereological methods for morphometric cytology. J. Cell Biol. **30**, 23–48 (1966).

Weibel, E. R., Stäubli, W., Gnägi, H. R., Hess, F. A.: Correlated morphometric and biochemical studies on the liver cell. I. Morphometric model, stereologic methods and normal morphometric data for rat liver. J. Cell Biol. **42**, 68–91 (1969).

Wilson, J. W., Leduc, E.: Mitochondrial changes in the liver of essential fatty acid-deficient mice. J. Cell Biol. **16**, 281–296 (1963).

Windmueller, H. G.: An orotic acid-induced adenin reversed, inhibition of hepatic lipoprotein secretion in the rat. J. biol. Chem. **239**, 530–554 (1964).

Wooley, J. G., Sebrell, W. H.: Niacin (nicotinic acid), an essential growth factor for rabbits fed a purified diet. J. Nutr. **29**, 191–209 (1945).

Institute of Pathology, University of Hamburg
(Director: Prof. Dr. G. Seifert)

Insulitis—A Morphological Review

GÖTZ FREYTAG and GÜNTER KLÖPPEL

With 18 Figures

Contents

A. Introduction

The inflammatory infiltration of the islets of Langerhans in the human pancreas is one of the unusual findings in the histopathology of spontaneous diabetes mellitus. It is unusual because of its rarity, its relationship to diabetes and its theoretical significance for the pathogenesis of the disease. The Zurich pathologist H. von Meyenburg coined the term "insulitis" because of the specific localization of the inflammation. The comparatively rare cases of an insulitis in post-mortem examinations of diabetics are in contrast to the great number of cases with uncharacteristic changes. The occurrence of insulitis has thus far been limited to juvenile diabetics who died shortly after the onset of their disease. This group of diabetics, however, seems to develop insulitis very regularly as stated by Gepts (1965). It has never been observed in chronic juvenile and adult diabetics (see addendum p. 36!). In contrast to the remarkable changes in the islets, such as insular hyalinosis and fibrosis, which are seen both in diabetics and also sporadically in non-diabetics, insulitis can be considered a specific histopathological manifestation of diabetes mellitus. Furthermore, since insulitis is typically found soon after the onset of the disease, it has considerable influence on the concept about the etiology and pathogenesis of diabetes in man. In origin it is particularly thought to be an infectious, degenerative, immunological or multifactorial phenomenon. The morphological contribution therefore tries to call attention to those changes in the islets which may either confirm or oppose one of these theories. The discussion of the histopathological findings also takes into consideration clinical, biochemical and serologic data presently available for diabetes. Furthermore, the discussion of this problem relies on experimental observations since insulitis can be induced in animals in different ways. Inflammation of the islet tissue occurs in some species after active immunization with insulin, as well as after injection of anti-insulin serum. Furthermore, islet infiltrates are described in experimental infections with certain viruses. The morphological substrate of these different experimental models of insulitis is not uniform but is always restricted to the endocrine portion of the pancreas. Thus this type of inflammation of the pancreas is easily distinguishable from that produced by inflammation of the exocrine tissue. Based on intensive studies of insulitis in animal models, autoimmune mechanisms are widely considered to play a role in the development of insulitis in juvenile diabetes.

Originally the term insulitis was used solely to characterize the lymphocytic infiltration of the islets of Langerhans in diabetics. The use of the term is still often restricted to this particular finding, with its cytologic particularity. Experimental studies, however, have revealed that besides a lymphocytic type of insulitis, there are acute insular infiltrates consisting mainly of granulocytes. The coexistence of both types of changes in the islets can also be observed. A strict separation of a "true" insulitis from other types of insular infiltrates contradicts the principles of general pathology: the term insulitis is thus used for all infiltrates localized within or around the islets without any relation to their cytological character. Insulitis can therefore have a lymphocytic, histiocytic or granulocytic pattern. On the basis of the experimental parallels, the eosinophilic infiltration around the islets in pancreata of infants of diabetic mothers will also be classed as insulitis.

B. Insulitis in Man

I. Specific Occurrence of Insulitis in Diabetes Mellitus

Since the classic experiment of v. MERING and MINKOWSKY (1889), characteristic histopathological changes of the pancreatic islets of diabetics are
expected. When morphological research into diabetes began, findings were
described in great number (SSOBOLEFF, 1902; SAUERBECK, 1902; OPIE, 1910;
WEICHSELBAUM, 1910 and 1911; HEIBERG, 1910 and 1911). The first definite
histopathology of the islets of Langerhans was given by WEICHSELBAUM (1910
and 1911). Later, the histological experiences from numerous autopsies of
diabetics showed that over all, only small changes of the islet system exist.
In particular, there is no correlation between the extent of the islet alterations
and the clinical and biochemical data. This finding primarily concerns the most
widespread diabetes in adults, for which no specific alterations of the islets
are found. As a morphological substrate most frequently noted in older diabetics, insular hyalinosis is observed in 45 % to 50 % of all cases (WARREN
et al., 1966). However, islet hyalinization is also reported in 4 % to 10 % of
nondiabetics (GEPTS, 1957; SEIFERT, 1958). The findings in juvenile-onset
diabetes, on the other hand, are more uniform. After a long run of the disease
a quantitative reduction of the islet tissue is often observed. MACLEAN and
OGILVIE (1955 and 1959), SEIFERT (1958) and GEPTS (1965) reported a decrease
in number and size of the islets. Even if normal islets are present, the number
of the beta cells is reduced. Thus, GEPTS (1965) showed by means of morphometric methods that the number of beta cells is considerably lower in diabetics
who died within six months after the onset of their disease (100 to 1000 per cm^2
of pancreatic tissue) than in controls (1000–10.000 per cm^2 of pancreatic tissue).
The relative proportion of the alpha cells in Langerhans islets increases with
the reduction of the beta cells, and this relative increase expresses itself in a
displacement of the alpha-beta cell ratio (TERBRÜGGEN, 1948; HULTQUIST et
al., 1948; FERNER, 1952; CREUTZFELDT and THEODOSSIO, 1957; GEPTS, 1957;
SEIFERT, 1958). Lymphocytic infiltration of the pancreatic islets was found
only in juvenile diabetics who died soon after the clinical onset of their disease.
It is regarded as a specific but rare finding in diabetes, when the frequency of
this disease is considered. However, if only the acute cases of juvenile diabetes
are taken into consideration, an inflammation of the endocrine pancreas is
seen in about 70 % of the cases (GEPTS, 1965). The autopsy material studied
by WARREN et al. (1966) revealed a similar frequency of insulitis. Eleven
patients in whom the onset of diabetes occurred below the age of 30 were
examined. Generally, diabetes had run a rapid course, too. An insulitis was
observed in eight of these cases.

II. History

An inflammatory infiltration of the islets of Langerhans was described
by the first workers on histopathology of diabetes (OPIE, 1901; SCHMIDT,

4*

1902; Cecil, 1909; Heiberg, 1911; Fischer, 1915). The observations known at that time were reviewed and completed with his own findings by Kraus, in his handbook article of 1929. These included: atrophy following hydropic degeneration, simple atrophy and hyaline degeneration. He described "chronic peri- and intra-insular inflammation (islet sclerosis)" as the fourth type of islet changes in association with diabetes mellitus. The literature of that time also shows that round cell infiltrates of the pancreatic islets are predominantly confined to cases suffering from infantile diabetes. Schmidt (1902) and Fischer (1915) reported a strongly marked infiltration of the islets by lymphocytes in children aged 6 and 10. Heiberg (1911) found mono-nucleated cell infiltrates which were variably pronounced in the islet area and in one case affected only single islets in infants with diabetes mellitus.

According to Weichselbaum (1910) the majority of the early investiga-tors of diabetes regarded the lymphocytic infiltrates in the islets as evidence for the degenerative—inflammatory etiology of the islet destruction. The term "islet sclerosis" established by Kraus (1929) for the chronic peri- and intrainsular inflammation makes the point that island destruction is based on progressive increase of the interstitial tissue of the islets due to degenera-tive processes. Thus, atrophy of the islets, as well as "productive inflammation" in juvenile diabetes, was regarded as a uniform mechanism of beta-cell degenera-tion. Only Heiberg (1911) and Fischer (1911) suggested that round cell infiltration represented a real inflammation. The discussion about the patho-genetic significance of the lymphocytic islet infiltrates ends in the review by Kraus (1929) with the statement: "After all, the question about the signifi-cance of the lymphocytic invasion of the islets has only little importance for the origin of diabetes." In the English literature, specially Warren (Warren and Root, 1925; Warren, 1927; Stansfield and Warren, 1928) referred in several papers to the islet infiltration as a specific finding in post-mortem examinations of juvenile diabetics. The report by Stansfield and Warren (1928) describing two children aged 12 and 15 who died, despite intensive insulin therapy, in diabetic coma, is particularly instructive. In the one case diabetes had run five days, in the other a few weeks. The pancreatic islets of both children were strongly invaded by round mononucleated cells. Le Compte (1958) described four cases of diabetes in infants and in juvenile patients aged eleven months, nine and seventeen years, respectively who died a few days after the clinical onset of the disease and showed insulitis at autopsy. In one of them, in addition to lymphocytes and monocytes, granulocytes were observed to a greater extent in the islets. Another observation of insulitis in a juvenile diabetic was reported by Nagler and Taylor (1963). Recently, two patients with lymphocytic insulitis were examined by Steiner (1968). The report deals with the findings in two infantile diabetics in whom the disease had also run a rapid course. Both children, an infant aged nine months and a child aged 2 years, died within one week after the onset of the first clinical symptoms. Some granulocytes were found amongst the inflammatory cells of the insular infiltrate, although the dominating cells were small lym-

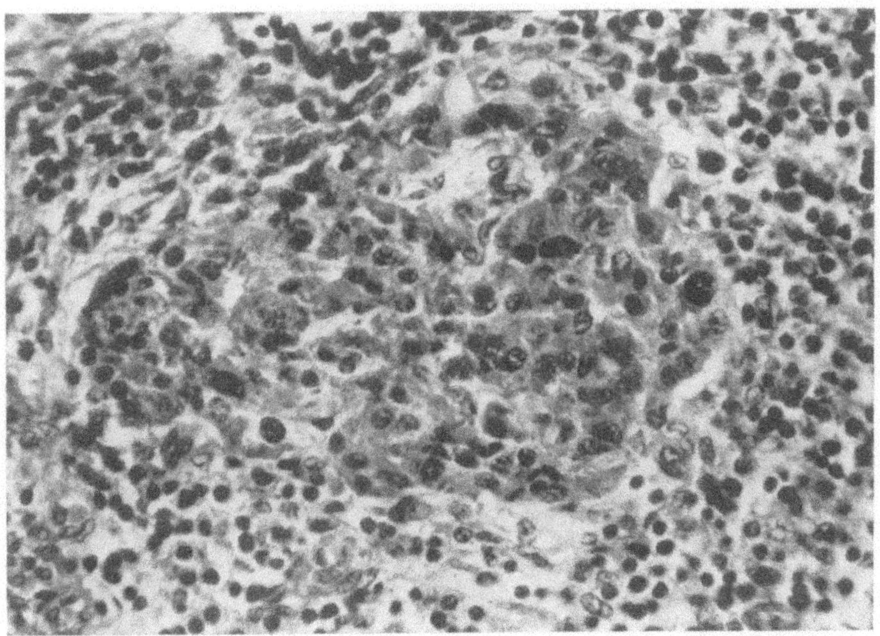

Fig. 1. Insulitis in a patient with juvenile diabetes of short duration. Extensive infiltration of small and some large lymphocytic cells mainly around the islet. Beta cells often show hypertrophy and irregular shape of the nucleus. PAS. × 500

phocytes. In an extensive study of this islet lesion in diabetes, GEPTS (1965) examined 22 cases of juvenile diabetes and found insulitis in 68 %. The duration of the disease ranged from 3 to 180 days. The age of the patients ranged from 12 months to 22 years. Except for three patients above the age of 18, nearly all others showing insulitis were infants. Insulitis was absent in only two patients aged 15; however, one of them showed a marked islet fibrosis. As mentioned above, the study emphasizes that insulitis, in contrast to the generally held view, is almost a common lesion, if one takes into consideration only juvenile diabetics whose disease follows an acute course.

III. Histopathology

It can be shown from most of the reports mentioned above, that the round mononucleated cells are predominantly localized around the islets, while intra-insular infiltration is less marked (Fig. 1). Incidentally, the directly adjoining acinous tissue is also invaded by a small number of inflammatory cells (WEICHSELBAUM, 1920; STANSFIELD and WARREN, 1928; LE COMPTE, 1958; WARREN et al. 1966). STEINER (1968) emphasizes that islets localized around pancreatic ducts, so-called duct islets, are frequently involved. As noted in all reports, the inflammatory infiltrate consists predominantly of small lymphocytes. Occasionally, large mononucleated cells have also been observed (STANSFIELD and WARREN, 1928; LE COMPTE, 1958). GEPTS (1965) described these

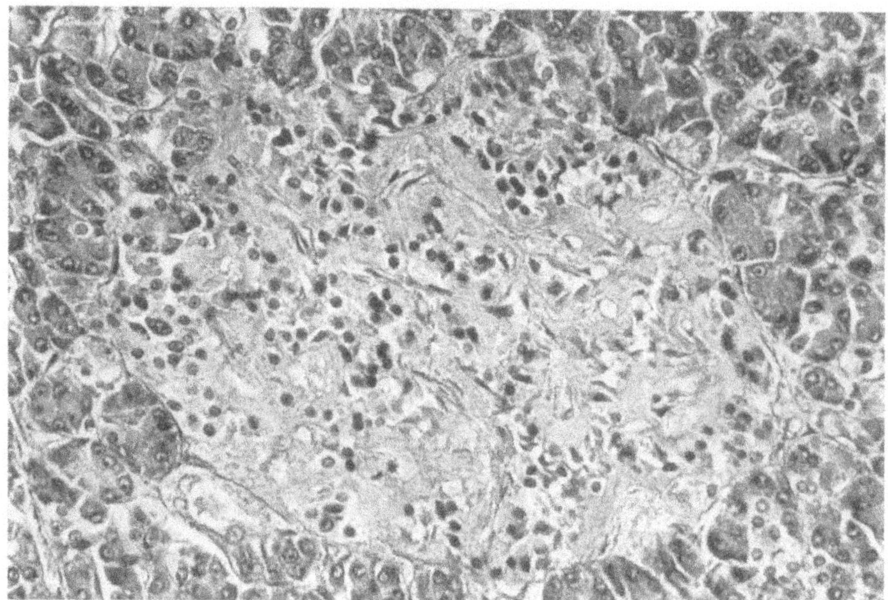

Fig. 2. Extensive fibrosis of pancreatic islet in a juvenile diabetic aged 15 years. Note the remaining cords of small insular cells (alpha cells? atrophic beta cells?). PAS. × 300

large mononucleated cells as reticulum cells. Granular leukocytes have been noted only in single incidences (Gepts, 1965; Warren *et al.*, 1966; Steiner, 1968). All authors, however, emphasize the lack of plasma cells in the cytology of the inflammation. The changes of the beta cells of the affected islets are not uniform. In the cases reported by Gepts (1965), islets of type II were most frequently infiltrated by lymphoid cells. Histologically this islet type seems to characterize the early phase of juvenile diabetes (Gepts, 1965). Often these islets are considerably enlarged and consist of swollen beta cells showing heavy degranulation. These islets are in general sharply outlined against the exocrine tissue of the pancreas. In individual cases lymphocytic infiltrates were also observed around islets of type I which were usually small and consisted of cords of small insular cells (Gepts, 1965) representing possibly alpha cells and atrophic beta cells. In addition, these islets often showed some degree of fibrosis (Fig. 2). Islets of type III, representing normal islets, have never been seen in connection with insulitis. According to some authors, the islets of type II characterize a compensating hypertrophy of remaining islet tissue during progressive deterioration of beta cells. The occasional formation of central cavities lined with cylindrical or cuboid epithelial cells in the islets of type II is regarded—by Gepts (1965)— as a sign of islet neoformation by proliferation of duct epithelium or centroacinar cells. The secretory hyperactivity of the beta cells in islets of type II is represented by cellular enlargement, an almost complete degranulation and, in some instances, a hydropic degeneration. Further characteristic features of the secretory hyperactivity are hypertrophy and irregular shape of numerous nuclei. These nuclear anomalies have been observed only in juvenile diabetes of short duration. Moreover, the observation of the so-called Weichselbaum corpuscles probably constitutes evidence of an enhanced insulin synthesis. These corpuscles have vague outlines and, when stained, exhibit behavior different from that of the secretory granules of the beta cells. They appear as a washed-out grey-blue when stained with hematoxylin, as blue when stained with toluidine blue and as red when stained with pyronine. In contrast to the secretory granules, these corpuscles are very sensitive to digestion with ribonuclease. Thus GEPTS (1965) suggested that they represent an increase of cytoplasmic ribonucleins in the hypertrophic beta cells. Their pathognomonic significance still remains to be clarified. Nevertheless, it is likely that they represent a hyperplasia of the rough endoplasmic reticulum due to enhanced protein synthesis.

IV. Pathogenesis and Etiology

The etiology of insulitis in man and its association with diabetes mellitus still remain unclear. Various pathogenic factors have been discussed with regard to the possible origin of the insulitis, i.e. reaction to beta cell damage by
1) infectious agents
2) toxic agents
3) functional overstimulation
4) immunologic mechanisms.

1. Infectious Agents

The hypothesis of an infectious etiology of insulitis is based on the observation that in some cases the onset of diabetes is closely connected in time to a preceding feverish infection (JOHN, 1949; FARRELL et al., 1953; BROWN, 1956). In particular, infectious viruses are presumed to be the etiological agents (GAMBLE et al., 1969). Among the viral diseases, some authors suggest that mumps may have an etiologic significance for the development of diabetes mellitus (BARBIERI, 1909; GUNDERSEN, 1927; KREMER, 1947; MELIN and URSING, 1958). GUNDERSEN (1927) described a remarkable increase of diabetes during the years following epidemic parotitis in Norway. MELIN and URSING (1958) could show in catamnestic studies that in forty children diabetes had developed a short time after the manifestion of an epidemic parotitis. In recent years attention has been drawn to infection with group B coxsackie viruses and its possible association with diabetes, since high antibody titers against these viruses have been detected in a significant number of diabetics (GAMBLE et al., 1969). These data led to the assumption that the onset of diabetes may be caused by an infection with coxsackie viruses. In animals, occurrence of diabetes due to viral infections have been documented. The passage of coxsackie viruses in adult mice has been shown to involve the pancreas (PAPPENHEIMER et al., 1951). BARBONI and MANOCCHIO (1962) reported a manifestation of diabetes in cattle recovering from foot-and-mouth disease (aphtous virus). Lymphocytic infiltrates in the pancreas of the diabetic cows have sometimes been observed in the vicinity of the islets. Müntefering *et al.* (1971) as well as Craighead and Steinke (1971) reported similar findings in mice infected with the M variant of the encephalomyocarditis virus. The pancreata of these mice exhibited necrotizing lesions of beta cells after the third day of the study. During the second and third week, moreover, infiltrates within and adjacent to the islets, consisting of mononuclear cells and granulocytes, were observed in some animals. Such morphological findings, together with the occurrence of a diabetic syndrome, suggest that this virus multiples particularly in the pancreatic islet cells, although the viral agent has not yet been identified in the beta cells.

As for diabetes in man, in the majority of patients, no clear evidence is available for an infectious origin of the disease. The few cases supporting the viral genesis of insulitis, and accordingly of diabetes mellitus, are offset by the predominantly greater number of diabetics in whom anamnestically no viral infection could be revealed. However, it is still conceivable that viral infection plays a role in the development of diabetes, particularly, if one combines it with genetic factors. From this point of view diabetes may be due to an inborn defect in mechanisms which are required for the replacement of diseased beta cells (Craighead and Steinke, 1971).

2. Toxic Beta Cell Damage

In addition to infection and destruction of the islet cells by viruses, damage by cytotoxic agents with great specificity are discussed. Degenerative alterations of the beta cells are always observed together with the finding of inflammatory infiltration of the islets. The hypothesis of beta cell damage by as yet unknown toxins was discussed by Le Compte (1958). He assumed that toxic beta cell damage would cause inflammatory cells to accumulate, followed later by an increase of fibrous tissue. Bacterial toxins are well known to affect the metabolism of certain cells in some infections. Thus, a cytotoxic origin of certain inflammations of the heart, the liver and the kidney can be established. However, neither exogenous toxins nor cytotoxic substances in metabolic disorders producing specific beta cell damage have as yet been demonstrated in association with insulitis. That insulitis is minimally related to the destruction of beta cells is shown by the histologic picture of the pancreatic islets after administration of alloxan, diazoxide and streptozotocin, substances with strong beta cytotoxic properties. There are of course changes in the cytologic appearance and in the enzyme system of the beta cells after administration of these agents, but neither the application of toxic nor of subtoxic doses leads to an insulitis. The therapeutic administration of alloxan and diazoxide in patients with hormonally active islet cell adenomas is also not accompanied by inflammatory infiltrates, although mild damage of the islet cells may be observed. Sommers (1956) suggested that the agents leading to parenchymatous inflammation are not directed against the cells but against the basal membranes. The breaking down of basement membranes in various organs would then result in an aggregation of lymphocytes. However, no disruption of the basement membranes in the islets of juvenile diabetics with insulitis could be detected under a light microscope, even if there was some evidence of splitting of such membranes (LE COMPTE, 1958).

3. Functional Overstimulation

In addition to toxic damage of the islet tissue, degenerative alterations of the beta cells by functional overstimulation are considered to play a role in the development of insulitis. Functional overstimulation may, for example, be induced by a peripheral insulin resistance causing hyperinsulinism as seen in obesity. The idea that overstrain of the beta cells leads to insulitis was proposed by H. v. MEYENBURG (1940). He claimed that the aggregation of round mononucleated cells in insulitis implies an inflammatory, "resorptive reaction" on cells damaged by exhaustion. This theory, however, could be confirmed neither by experimental findings nor by observations in man. Although hyperinsulinism in spontaneously diabetic animals results in islet hyperplasia, insulitis has never yet been reported. Overproduction of the hormonal antagonists of insulin, as for example in Cushings' syndrome or acromegaly, is not accompanied by inflammatory infiltrates in and around the islets, despite marked signs of beta-cell hyperactivity. In these endocrine disorders the pancreatic islets can show complete degranulation and nuclear hypertrophy of the beta cells, similar to those findings described in acute juvenile diabetes. Insulitis, however, never occurs. The same histologic results are obtained under experimental conditions when diabetes is induced by long-term treatment with growth hormone (VOLK and LAZARUS, 1963). Young animals, in particular, then show a pronounced mitotic rate in the beta cells and a neogenesis of the islets, whereas lymphocytic infiltrates in the pancreas are lacking.

4. Immunological Mechanisms of Insulitis

In recent years it has been emphasized that immunological mechanisms as primary pathogenic factors may account for the development of an insulitis. In this regard, it is of particular interest to note that experimental insulitis, morphologically resembling the lymphocytic islet infiltration in acute-onset juvenile diabetes, can be induced by active immunization with insulin (RENOLD et al., 1964; TORESON et al., 1964). The histologic feature of both experimental and human insulitis is in accordance with an immunological reaction of the cellular type observed in delayed hypersensitivity, whereas it cannot be compared with the inflammatory infiltrate due to an immune reaction of the immediate type. In addition, specific localization of this inflammatory process gave rise to a discussion of these changes on the basis of immunological mechanisms specifically directed against the islets.

If we assume that an autoimmune process plays an important role in the pathogenesis of this islet lesion, a sensitization of immune cells against specific proteins of the beta cells has to be considered. Viral and genetic mechanisms are discussed as factors which may induce antigenicity of autologous proteins. Multifactoral genesis has also been emphasized. Under these hypothetical points of view the following observations can now be reviewed.

Based on their own observations of insulitis, Solomon and Blizzard (1963) suggested an immunological etiology of the "idiopathic diabetes mellitus", drawing the histopathological parallel between the insulitis and the findings in other endocrine and nonendocrine diseases for which an autoimmune mechanism is very likely. Furthermore, clinical observations and serological results pointing to an apparent association between diabetes and diseases characterized by organ-specific autoimmunity provide some evidence for a general autoimmune reactivity in diabetics. Thus Stanton et al. (1954) regarded the remarkable syntropy of diabetes with the idiopathical type of Addison's disease as an indication of a common autoimmune disorder. In this regard, the study of Beaven et al. (1959) also demands attention, since a concomitance of diabetes, Addison's disease and Hashimoto's thyroiditis has been established. An extensive report summarizing the clinical data of this endocrine syndrome, sometimes called Schmidt's syndrome, was given by Carpenter et al. (1964). Landing et al. (1963) frequently found thyroid antibodies in juvenile-onset diabetics. Moore and Neilson (1963) concluded from their studies that gastric complement-fixing antibodies were also significantly more common in juvenile diabetics. Irvine et al. (1970) found an increased incidence of antibodies to thyroid cytoplasm and to gastric parietal cell cytoplasm in young insulin-dependent diabetics. The incidence of these antibodies was independent of the duration of the diabetes, so the phenomenon seems not to be secondary to diabetes. These authors therefore suggested that diabetes is associated with disturbed immunity, which both may be due to a common genetic fault. Steiner (1968), on the other hand, refused the hypothesis of a general "autoimmune diathesis". Because of the apparent beta cell disappearance, he assumed that a specific autoimmune disorder, possibly produced by an infection as a "basic noxa", may involve the beta cell system as a whole, leading in time to an absolute beta cell deficiency. Evidence for cellular hypersensitivity against pancreatic components, possibly of cytoplasmic origin, has recently been given by Nerup et al. (1971). They demonstrated an organspecific species-nonspecific, antipancreatic hypersensitivity in treated and untreated diabetics against extracts from porcine pancreata, by means of the leukocyte migration test and an intracutaneous testing. The extract was prepared by homogenization and differential centrifugation from pooled porcine pancreata in which atrophy of the exocrine tissue had been induced by ligation of the pancreatic duct. The studies showed also that the insulin content of the preparations cannot be held responsible for the immune reaction. It remains therefore to be clarified whether the antigenic components belong to the beta cell system at all.

If one considers an autoimmune disorder against the insulin-producing system, the mechanism by which the beta cells may become antigenic has then to be explained. STEINER (1968) offered the hypothesis that viruses possibly play a role. For example, it is conceivable that viruses induce faulty synthesis of proteins by alteration of the DNA structure during multiplication in the beta cells. These altered proteins are then considered antigens by the immune system. On the other hand, it can be suggested, on the basis of genetic predisposition to diabetes, that structural changes in insulin or associated proteins occur, thus resulting in antigenicity. Furthermore, as suggested by IRVINE et al. (1970), a general disturbance of immunological tolerance, due to viral infection or to a polygenic predisposition, must also be considered. Lastly, there might be an association or an interdependence between viral infection, inherited factors and immune mechanisms at the onset of diabetes. Genetic defects of the beta cell, as for example defects of membranes, insulin release, insulin biosynthesis or reproduction of beta cells, may support the destruction of these cells by viruses, which then results in a rapid functional collapse. When this occurs, immunological mechanisms can be elicited by altered proteins (FREYTAG, 1973).

These theories attempt to summarize the main concepts regarding participation of autoimmune mechanisms in the origin of insulitis and juvenile diabetes. As for adult-onset diabetes, characterized by its slow course, these ideas are, however, hardly appropriate. In opposition to the multifactoral concept of juvenile diabetes, diabetes in adults may therefore only be caused by the manifestation of a single inborn defect in connection with certain environmental factors.

Since autoimmune factors appeared to be important for the development of juvenile diabetes, an intensive search for circulating insulin antibodies has been carried out. Various serologic, electrophoretic and fluorescence microscopic techniques have been employed. Most of the studies, however, have been unsuccessful. Positive results have been reported only by PAV et al. (1963), MANCINI et al. (1964, 1965), CHETTY and WATSON (1965) and PENCHEV et al. (1968). PAV et al. (1963) and CHETTY and WATSON (1965) reported complement fixation in the presence of insulin in untreated diabetics. MANCINI et al. (1964 and 1965) demonstrated antibodies against human insular tissue in the serum of untreated diabetics by means of fluorescence microscopy. PENCHEV et al. (1968) found precipitating antibodies to insulin in 20 % of untreated diabetics. Despite these findings, the presence of antibodies to insulin or to other components of the beta cells is still to be confirmed. Furthermore, it is necessary to mention the studies of ROY et al. (1968), who suggested by their experiments the existence of an "abnormal" insulin in diabetics, characterized by a stronger resistance to insulinase.

It can thus be stated that in spite of extensive studies, an autoimmune genesis of diabetes on the basis of genetic or infectious factors has not yet been confirmed, and remains purely hypothetic. Lymphocytic infiltration of the islets resembling human insulitis can be induced in animals under certain conditions, but it is unknown whether these experimental models are also valid for the etiology of insulitis in man. In the following chapters (D, E) insulitis-inducing experiments will be described in detail.

Addendum. Recent observations [Le Compte, P. M., Legg, M. A.: Insulitis (Lymphocytic Infiltration of Pancreatic Islets) in Late-onset Diabetes. Diabetes 21, 762 1971] in two patients with late-onset diabetes revealed an insulitis of pancreatic islets. This indicates that insulitis is not restricted to juvenile diabetics but can also occur in patients with maturity-onset diabetes. Studies to demonstrate cell-bound antibodies by immunofluorescent techniques or to recover a virus from pancreas in these cases were unsuccesful.

C. Acute Eosinophilic Insulitis in Infants of Diabetic Mothers

I. Histopathology and History

Inflammatory infiltration of the pancreatic islets observed exclusively in infants of diabetic mothers can be separated from destructive insulitis in juvenile diabetics. The difference in the histological features, in relation to the lymphocytic insulitis described above, is characterized by the great number of eosinophilic granulocytes. Mononucleated cells as well as neutrophilic granulocytes can also be observed but are in general more rare. The cellular infiltrates often spread out in the peri-insular and interacinar spaces in certain parts of the pancreas whereas other areas are not infiltrated. The stromatic infiltration is not sharply outlined against the surrounding interacinar spaces. Besides the inflammatory changes, hypertrophy and hyperplasia of the islets and the single beta cells are obvious (Fig. 3). Dubreuil and Anderoidas (1920) were the first to point out that hypertrophy and an increase in the number of islets in the fetus are frequently associated with maternal diabetes. Van Beek (1939), who particularly called attention to the significance of the insular hyperplasia in infants of diabetic mothers, described giant islets with heavy degranulated beta cells. This finding was repeatedly confirmed later on (Helwig, 1940; Cardell, 1953). On the other hand the polymorphocellular infiltrates attracted attention for the first time when they were described by Warren and Le Compte (1952), who presumed that this finding might represent extramedullary hematopoiesis in the pancreas, since it occurs in liver and spleen in erythroblastosis fetalis. Seven infants of diabetic mothers were examined histochemically and histologically by McKay *et al.* (1953). The pancreata of these infants showed insular hyperplasia as well as peri-insular and interacinar infiltrates. It is noteworthy that only the largest islets were surrounded by eosinophiles, neutrophiles and some mononuclear cells such as lymphocytes and monocytes. In addition, Charcot-Leyden crystals could be demonstrated in almost all cases. Driscoll *et al.* (1960) stated that insular hyperplasia is frequently associated with infiltration. They found that the

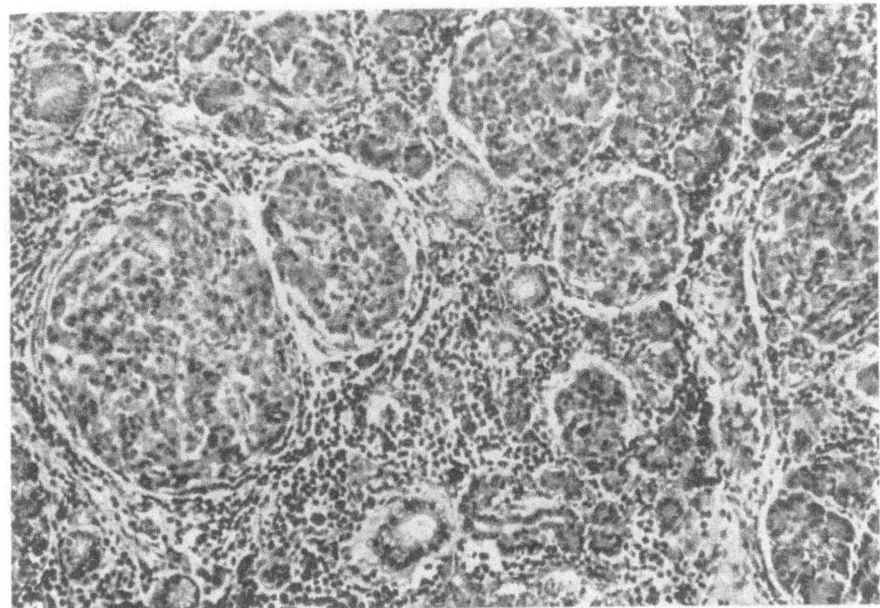

Fig. 3. Hyperplasia of pancreatic islets in newborn of diabetic mother. Note the extensive granulocytic infiltrate around the islets, extending into the adjacent interacinar spaces. Giemsa stain. × 180

degree of insular hyperplasia was greatest in the largest babies but that it was independent of the severity of the maternal diabetes or of the time of survival of the babies. This was stated previously by VAN BEEK (1939) who showed that the pancreatic changes are not related to the course and the severity of the diabetic disease in the mother. D'AGOSTINO and BAHN (1963) noted a diffuse interstitial fibrosis of the pancreas in association with the cellular infiltration which they interpreted as presumptive evidence of a subacute form of interstitial pancreatitis.

II. Pathogenesis and Etiology

In principle, the same factors are discussed for the etiology and pathogenesis of insulitis in infants of diabetic mothers as were reviewed for insulitis in juvenile diabetics. A viral genesis has, indeed, never been suggested. VAN BEEK (1939) interpreted the cellular infiltrates as a consequence of the degeneration which appeared to her to be a result of functional overstrain. She therefore presumed that the islets of infants in diabetic and prediabetic mothers which have been overstrained during pregnancy are not able to cope with the increasing stress of life after birth. Diabetes mellitus would then develop on the basis of the previous islet damage. In addition to this "exogenous" islet damage during the prenatal period, a genetic factor is also suggested in the pathogenesis of diabetes. McKAY et al. (1953) claimed that functional overstrain of the single beta cell in the fetal islet may perhaps result in a release of altered islet proteins or even an insulin precursor leading to an inflammatory reaction.

Evidence of hyperactivity of the endocrine pancreas during the fetal period is undoubtedly provided by morphological investigation, as the intensive studies by Silverman (1963), Borchard and Müntefering (1969) and Van Assche (1968, 1970) have shown in recent years. The correlation between birth weight and insular hyperplasia has also been prooved to be statistically significant. However, it is totally unknown which factor might induce the development of giant islets. The hypoglycemia often observed post partum in newborns of diabetic mothers implies that there is indeed a hyperinsulinismus. Hypoglycemic reaction in infants is more marked when high maternal blood sugar levels are measured before delivery (Pedersen, 1952; Baird and Farquhar, 1962). Moreover, an increased insulin content in the whole pancreas was found in infants of diabetic mothers (Steinke and Driscoll, 1965). Maternal hyperglycemia has until now been regarded as an important factor in stimulating the fetal beta cell system during pregnancy, since it would cause an excessive supply of glucose in fetal circulation. On the other hand, the properties of human placental lactogen hormone in stimulating insulin release have recently been demonstrated. This hormone originates from the placenta and, as regards its effect on metabolism, exhibits behavior similar to that of the growth hormone (Spellacy, 1969 and 1971). Improvement of the maternal diabetes by insulin production in the fetus, as formerly suggested, does not occur since insulin does not appear to pass through the placental barrier in a biologically active form.

The clinical-histopathological study by Silverman (1963) took on great importance for the study of eosinophilic insulitis, because it clearly summarized the main data. By his systematic examinations, Silverman emphasized that the form of insulitis associated with insular hyperplasia occurs only in infants of diabetic or prediabetic mothers. The presence of stromatic and islet eosinophilia is not related to prior administration of exogenous insulin to the mother. There is no correlation between the degree of eosinophilic infiltrates, birth weight, length of gestation and hours of postnatal life. On the other hand, Silverman also demonstrated that islet hypertrophy is related mainly to birth weight. Because the stromatic and peri-insular infiltrates consisted mainly of eosinophilic granulocytes, Silverman suggested that this finding may represent the occurrence of an immune mechanism within the islets. If an immune reaction is involved it is unlikely that insulitis in infants is induced by immunization with a fetal antigen, since the number of pregnancies is not related to the extent of the inflammation in the pancreata of the individual infants. Moreover, experimental studies point to a failure of transplacental insulin transport from the fetus to the mother (Davies and Lacy, 1957). Therefore if stromatic eosinophilia and eosinophilic insulitis are based on immunological mechanisms, it is more conceivable that these changes are due to maternal antibodies against autologous insulin which also react with the fetal insulin. Maternal immunoglobulins and fetal insulin may then form antigen-antibody complexes which are known to elicit a leuko-tactic process (COCHRAN and DIXON, 1968). This is shown by the specific localization and the eosinophilic nature of the infiltrate. The demonstration of antibodies against the Rh-factor in infants with fetal erythroblastosis clearly shows that diaplacental transport of IgG-antibodies is possible. Acquired insulin antibodies do not play a role in this phenomenon, since inflammatory infiltrates were also observed in infants of diabetic mothers who had never been treated with exogenous insulin.

Experimentally, similar infiltrates consisting of eosinophilic and neutrophilic granulocytes as well as some mononuclear cells occur within and around the islets of mice and rats injected with anti-insulin serum from guinea pigs (LACY et al., 1963; LACY and WRIGHT, 1965; FREYTAG et al., 1969; KLÖPPEL et al., 1971). The characteristic parallels between the pattern of the inflammatory infiltrate after administration of insulin-antibodies and the histopathological feature arising from a locally induced Arthus phenomenon support the assumption that eosinophilic insulitis in infants of diabetic mothers is also elicited by an antigen-antibody reaction of the immediate type. Experimentally, the electron-microscopic observation of precipitated material adjacent to the beta cells after injection of anti-insulin serum demonstrates the presence of an antigen-antibody complex inducing insulitis under these conditions (KLÖPPEL et al., 1971).

D. Experimental Insulitis in Animals Immunized with Insulin

Active immunization with heterologous and homologous insulin results in the production of circulating antibodies in numerous species. A lymphocytic infiltration at the level of the pancreatic islets induced by immunization with insulin has, in contrast, so far only been demonstrated in cows, sheep and rabbits.

I. Experimental Insulitis in Cattle

The first observation of an experimental insulitis was purely accidental. RENOLD and co-workers (1964) immunized cattle with crystalline porcine and bovine insulin in Freund's adjuvant in order to study immunological responses to heterologous and homologous insulin. The immunization ran over six to 21 months, initially being carried out at two-week intervals, and later on at monthly intervals. One of the animals had to be killed after five months of immunization because it was strangled in its halter. Histological examination of the pancreas surprisingly revealed an inflammatory infiltration of the islets by mononucleated cells.

This histopathological finding was later confirmed in other animals (LE COMPTE et al., 1966). Four heifers immunized with insulin and two heifers immunized with Freund's adjuvant alone were examined histologically after a study lasting almost two years. One of the animals received bovine insulin, a second received porcine insulin, while the others first received bovine (porcine) and were later immunized with porcine (bovine) insulin. These four heifers showed a marked lymphocytic infiltration of the pancreatic islets, which was lacking in the controls. Often the normal islet architecture was completely destroyed by the infiltrates. In these islets beta cells, and perhaps alpha cells too, were definitely reduced in number. Besides the inflammatory infiltration some islets exhibited fibrosis with the complete absence of normal islet cells. The inflammatory cells were described as lymphocytes, predominantly of the "small" type and rarely of the "large" type, which invaded the islets to a variable extent. Histiocytes were not identified with certainty and plasma cells were notably absent. No specific finding of labeled bovine insulin or antibovine globulin antibody to the lymphocytic cells could be observed by fluorescence microscopy. The remaining beta cells showed signs of hyperactivity. The cytoplasm was degranulated and swollen and contained increased RNA, and the nuclei were enlarged. Since the total number of the beta cells was decreased, the extractable insulin of the pancreata was correspondingly reduced when compared with the controls. In spite of this evidence of impaired synthesis of insulin, no support for a diabetic state in these animals could be given by glucose tolerance tests.

In addition to the histological islet changes, immunization with heterologous (porcine) and homologous (bovine) insulin evoked antibodies in all heifers. The response to the heterologous porcine insulin was more rapid and more pronounced. In most cases nonprecipitating antibodies were produced which were able to decrease the hypoglycemic activity of injected exogenous insulin. A biological neutralization of endogenous insulin by an immunological binding could not be demonstrated with certainty.

II. Experimental Insulitis in Sheep

Similar serologic and histologic data were also obtained in sheep immunized with porcine or bovine insulin over six months to two years (Renold *et al.*, 1969). The islets showed marked lymphocytic infiltration. An insular fibrosis was already partially present. In addition, all animals had formed humoral antibodies to the injected insulin. The highest circulating titers of antibodies were observed in two sheep with the most marked insulitis. Besides this notable production of antibodies, pronounced delayed hypersensitivity tested by intracutaneous injections of insulin was also evident. When studied by fluorescence microscopy, labelled insulin appeared to be bound to leukocytes in the blood stream or in the area of the infiltrated islets (Federlin *et al.*, 1968).

III. Experimental Insulitis in Rabbits

As a third species, rabbits immunized with insulin frequently developed an insulitis (Toreson *et al.*, 1964). Some of the animals also showed a decreased tolerance of glucose or even an overt diabetes (GRODSKY *et al.*, 1966). In their first studies TORESON and co-workers (1964) noticed a striking hyperglycemia in two out of five rabbits after immunization with crystalline beef insulin in Freund's adjuvant. Moreover, in one case hyperglycemia was combined with an insulitis (GRODSKY *et al.*, 1966). During the first weeks of the experiment blood glucose levels rose to 400–600 mg/ml. One animal continued this extreme hyperglycemia until it died at twenty-one weeks, while the diabetic state of the other was still present, although improved, until the end of the study, which lasted sixty-two weeks. Antibody levels in these diabetic rabbits determined three to five weeks after the beginning of the immunization evidently exceeded those in the nondiabetic animals. On the contrary, the amounts of the total circulating bound insulin, at that time, were very small in the diabetic rabbits. Only later could an extremely high value be measured in the longest surviving animal in which diabetes had gradually improved. Histological examination of the pancreas of the nondiabetic animals revealed no marked alteration on the light- and electronmicroscopic levels when compared with controls. In the less severe diabetic rabbit, however, glycogen infiltration, extreme degranulation and hyperplasia of the endoplasmic reticulum of the beta cells were found in association with lymphocytic islet infiltration. In the other animal the islets showed no insulitis, but were atrophic and almost completely devoid of beta cells.

Further studies by these authors (TORESON *et al.*, 1968; LEE *et al.*, 1969) dealt with the influence of immunization procedures on developing an insulitis and with the pathogenetic classification of this islet lesion. Moreover, the relations between insulitis, circulating insulin antibody and hyperglycemia were examined. The mode of immunization leading to insulitis and hyperglycemia in rabbits corresponded with the methods normally used. The antigen was injected together with "complete" Freund's adjuvant, and later with "incomplete", at weekly intervals (ROBINSON and WRIGHT, 1961). Psittacosis agent and para-typhoid vaccine were employed as additional adjuvants to stimulate the production of antibodies to insulin. Their administration generally resulted in high antibody titers, but morphological effects were not reported. Single aggregates of mononuclear leukocytes in dilated capillaries of the pancreatic islets occurred in about one third of the rabbits one week after the first immunization with insulin in Freund's adjuvant. At this time no immunoreactive antibodies could be found. After the second immunization, many islets showed a pericapillary infiltration with mononuclear cells. Insulin antibodies were now evident while blood glucose was normal. The third immunization was followed by an extensive infiltration of the islets, associated with a reduction in the number of beta cells in two thirds of the animals. The infiltrating cells consisted of lymphocytes, macrophages and some plasma cells. Close contact between the mononuclear and the beta cells was frequently observed by electron microscopy. At this contact point, it appeared as if some of the beta cells would lose their cell membranes and release their cytoplasmic contents into the surrounding inter-

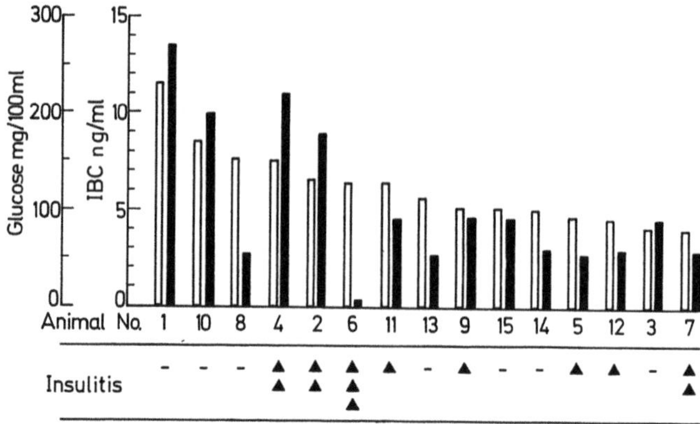

Fig. 4. Blood glucose levels, insulin binding capacity (IBC) and intensity and frequency of insulitis in rabbits 6 to 8 days after the four-weekly immunization with bovine insulin in Freund's adjuvant. □ Blood glucose level. ■ IBC, calculated on that dilution of serum with 50 % binding of 0.1 µg of porcine [127]J insulin/ml

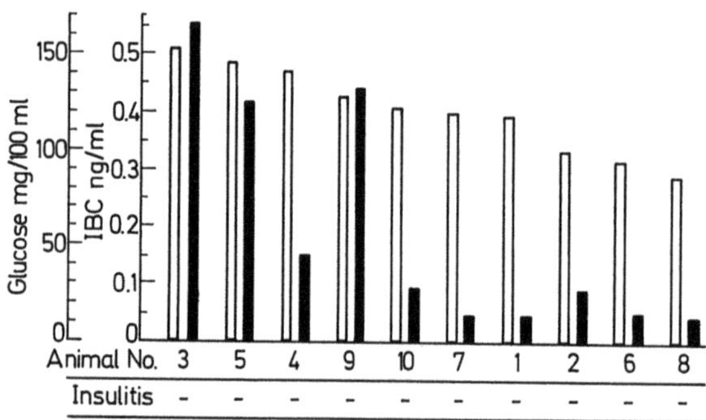

Fig. 5. Blood glucose levels, insulin binding capacity (IBC) and intensity and frequency of insulitis in rabbits 6 to 8 days after the four-weekly immunization with porcine insulin in Freund's adjuvant. □ Blood glucose level. ■ IBC, calculated on that dilution of serum with 50 % binding of 0.1 µg porcine [127]J insulin/ml

cellular spaces (Lee *et al.*, 1969). Studies by fluorescence microscopy of the pancreatic tissue exposed to labelled antirabbit gamma globulin sera or labelled bovine insulin were generally negative. Only plasma cells when present showed specific fluorescence after staining with labelled antirabbit gamma globulin sera.

The antibody titers usually reached maximum values three to four weeks after the first immunization. Transient hyperglycemias, on the average, appeared after four to seven weeks in the course of which the blood glucose levels rarely exceeded 300 mg/100 ml. Prolonged hyperglycemia or overt diabetes was only observed in a small number of instances. Attention was drawn to a correlation between the degree of insulitis and the incidence of hyperglycemia in some animals.

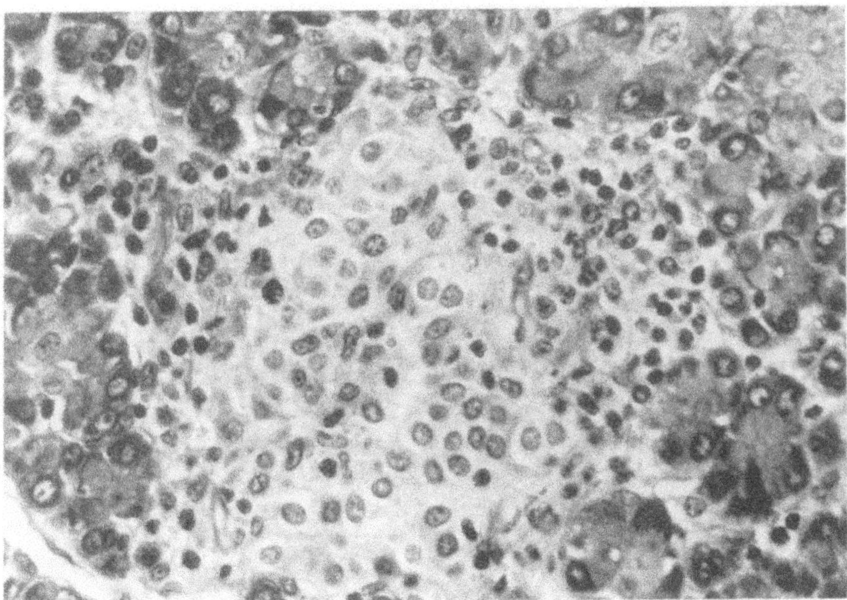

Fig. 6. Rabbit pancreas after weekly immunization with bovine insulin (4th week): Insulitis with round-cell infiltrates around the islet. Scattered lymphocytic cells are also present within the islet. PAS. × 500

In our own series of experiments (KLÖPPEL *et al.*, 1972), an insulitis was found in eight out of fifteen rabbits after four weeks immunization with bovine insulin in Freund's adjuvant. In contrast, no insulitis occurred after immunization with porcine insulin. Production of antibodies was observed in both groups of the study, but the antibody titers of the rabbits immunized with porcine insulin were in general much lower than the antibody titers in rabbits immunized with bovine insulin (Figs. 4 and 5). Antibody titer and hyperglycemia did not correlate with the incidence or even with the presence of insulitis (Fig. 4). Thus, the animal with the most marked insulitis remained normoglycemic and showed the lowest antibody titer, whereas maximum circulating antibody and highest blood glucose levels were measured in an animal without islet infiltration. In contrast, there was a general correlation in elevation of the blood glucose level and of the amount of the antibody titer in the single animals of both groups (Figs. 4 and 5). Rabbits in which the highest blood sugar levels had been recorded had on the average the highest antibody titers.

Under the light microscope, as mentioned briefly above (TORESON *et al.*, 1968; LEE *et al.*, 1969), insulitis in rabbits is characterized by an insular infiltrate consisting of mononuclear cells (Fig. 6). Sometimes, the inflammatory infiltration is observed only in single islets; sometimes, all islets are involved in the inflammatory process, which leads to a decomposition of the normal islet architecture. Under these circumstances, heavily destroyed islets contain only single beta cells surrounded by round mononucleated cells. The

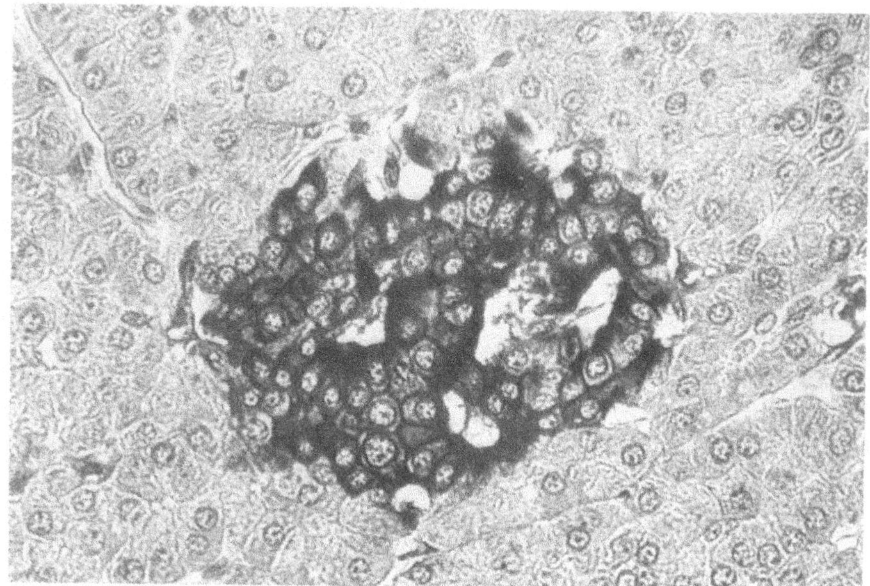

Fig. 7. a Normal rabbit islet with distinct granulation of the beta cells. Aldehyde fuchsin.
× 500. b Rabbit pancreas after weekly immunization with bovine insulin (4th week):
Peri- and intrainsular insulitis with marked destruction of islet. Degranulation, nuclear
hypertrophy and cytoplasmic hyperplasia of remaining beta cells. Aldehyde fuchsin.
× 500. (From Klöppel *et al.*, 1972)

remaining beta cells often show enlargement of nuclei and heavy degranulation as a sign of secretory hyperactivity (Fig. 7). Marked changes of the alpha cell structure are not evident. The islet infiltration often extends into the adja-

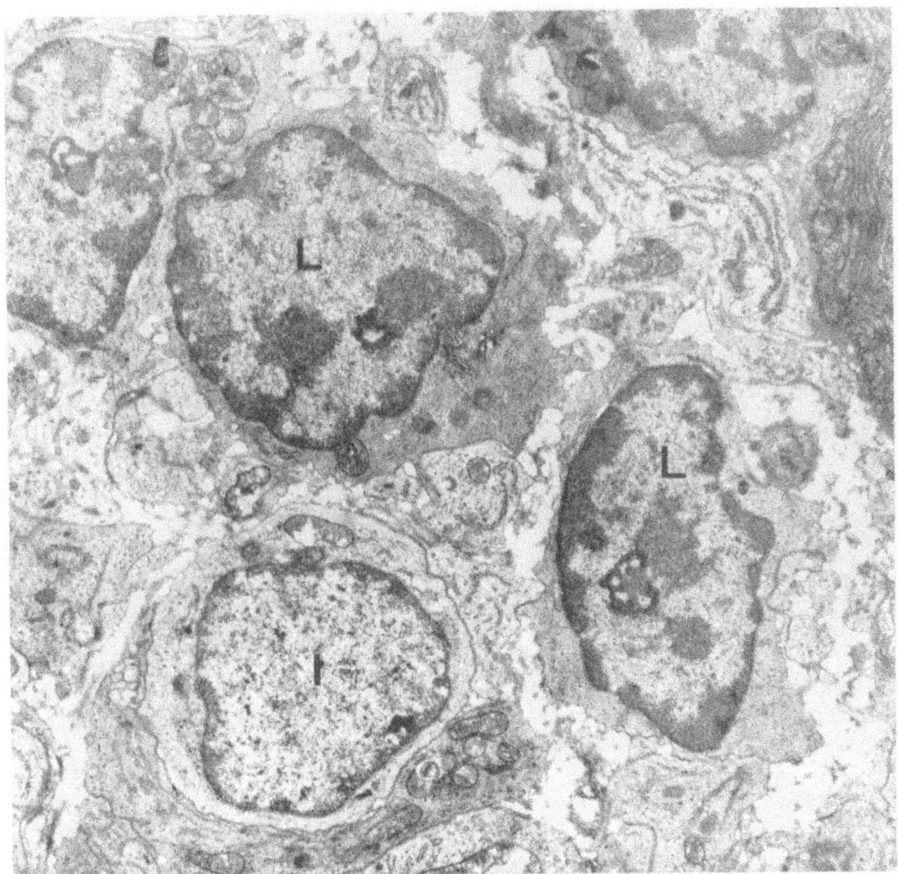

Fig. 8. Rabbit pancreas after weekly immunization with bovine insulin (4th week): Part of the peri-insular infiltrate. Several lymphocytes (*L*) of the intermediate type with well-developed nucleolus and abundant ribosomes in the cytoplasm. Nearby immunoblasts (*I*) with sparse granular cytoplasm and abundant cell organelles. × 7650. (From KLÖPPEL *et al.*, 1972)

cent acinous tissue. There the largest infiltrates of mononuclear cells are found around small veins and ducts. Under the electronmicroscope (TORESON *et al.*, 1968; LEE *et al.*, 1969; KLÖPPEL *et al.*, 1972) the infiltrating cells can be differentiated mainly as lymphocytes, lymphocytes of the intermediate type, and immunoblasts in different phases of development (Fig. 8). Plasma cells are rarely found beside these cell types, generally being located in the periphery of the infiltrate. Close contact between immune cells and beta cells is described as a usual occurrence. Moreover, the close approximation of these cells is frequently associated with a lysis of the adjacent cell membranes (Fig. 9). The ergastoplasm and the organelles of these affected beta cells are otherwise intact, or show a release of their cytoplasmic contents into the surrounding intercellular spaces. Other beta cells show degenerative changes (cystic dilatation of the endoplasmic reticulum and a shrinkage of the nucleus) although

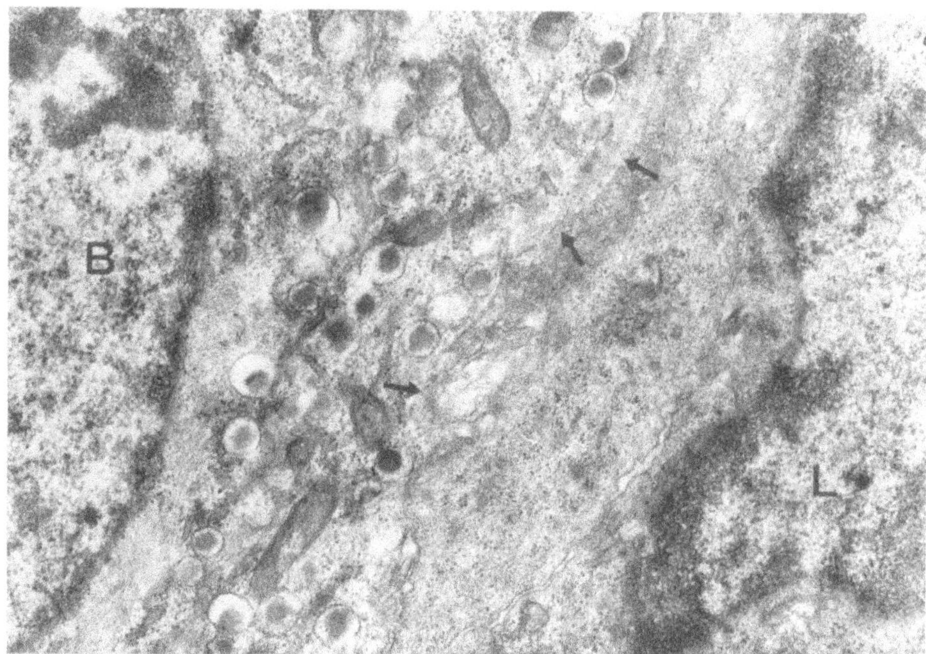

Fig. 9. Rabbit pancreas after weekly immunization with bovine insulin (4th week): Lymphocyte (*L*) in close contact to a bety cell (*B*). Circumscribed lysis of the cell membranes (↑). × 21 500. (From Klöppel *et al.*, 1972)

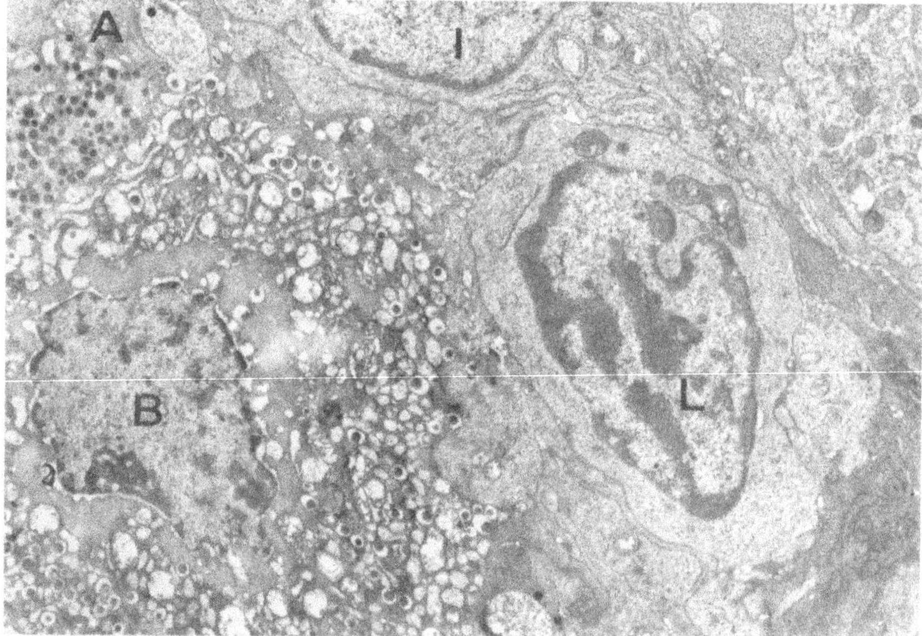

Fig. 10. Rabbit pancreas after weekly immunization with bovine insulin (4th week): Degenerative changes of a beta cell (*B*) with cystic dilatation of the rough endoplasmic reticulum and shrinkage of the nucleus. In the vicinity a lymphocyte (*L*) and an immunoblast (*I*). Alpha cell (*A*). × 6800. (From Klöppel *et al.*, 1972)

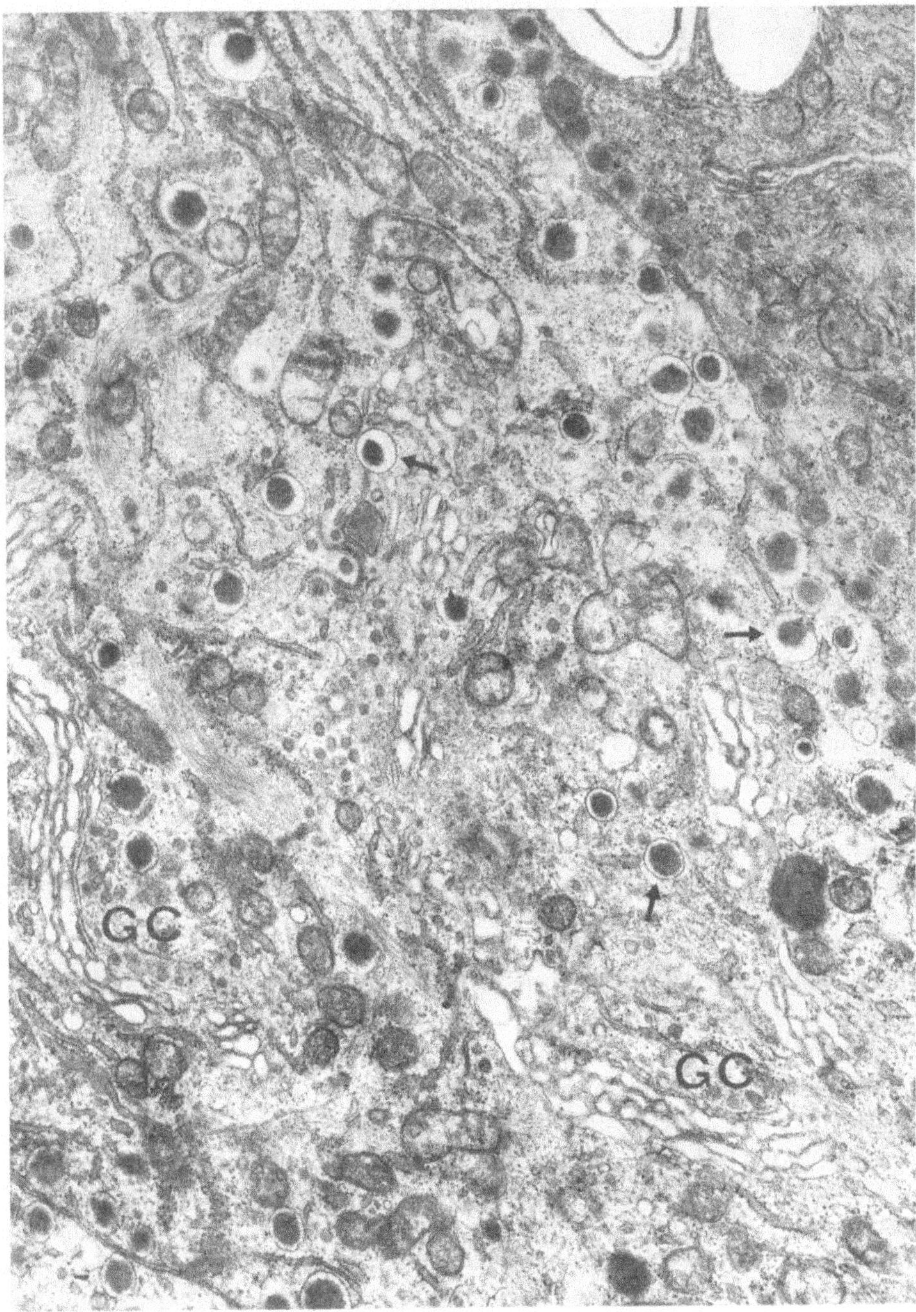

Fig. 11. Rabbit pancreas after weekly immunization with bovine insulin (4th week): Part of strongly activated beta cell of a rabbit with severe insulitis. Different electron dense granules (↑) and hyperplasia of the rough endoplasmic reticulum and the Golgi complexes (*GC*). In the vicinity of the Golgi complexes abundant microvesicles. × 19 500.
(From KLÖPPEL *et al.*, 1972)

the cell membranes appear to be undisturbed (Fig. 10). Sometimes, cellular debris is observed in macrophages. Lymphocytes and immunoblasts to some extent also have close contact with alpha cells and acinous cells. A small number of these acinous cells then show a focal degeneration of the cytoplasm. The still intact beta cells are often hyperactive, as indicated by an enlargement of the rough endoplasmic reticulum and the Golgi complexes (Volk et al., 1965). Furthermore, numerous microvesicles can be observed in the immediate vicinity of the Golgi apparatuses, and secretory granules are found in all stages of maturation (Fig. 11). In contrast, no remarkable changes of the beta cells occur in the rabbits without insulitis. Particularly, no remarkable signs of secretory hyperactivity of the beta cells are evident in hyperglycemic animals without insulitis.

IV. Pathogenesis and Etiology

As far as histological features and specific localization are concerned, insulitis in animals immunized with insulin and Freund's adjuvant suggests an immune response of the cellular type which has assumed an autoimmune character. Thus, the infiltrate at the level of the pancreatic islet consists mainly of lymphocytes and immunoblasts which are seen in delayed hypersensitivity. Eosinophilic and neutrophilic granulocytes characterizing an immune response of the immediate type are lacking. Similar findings by light- and electron-microscopy are observed in other experimental autoimmune disorders such as, for example, experimental thyroiditis (Witebsky et al., 1957; Weigle, 1965; Themann et al., 1968; Karesen, 1970), experimental parathyroiditis (Jankovic et al., 1965; Lupulescu, 1965), experimental adrenalitis (Colover and Glynn, 1958; Milcou et al., 1959) and experimental encephalomyelitis (Waksman and Adams, 1956; Waksmann, 1965). These experimental autoimmune disorders are induced by injections of homologous organ extracts or organ specific protein fractions together with Freund's adjuvant. Besides the formation of circulating antibodies, an organ specific lymphocytic infiltration is elicited in a large number of instances. Experimental thyroiditis, for example, is produced by sensitization of immune cells against extracted thyroglobulin, leading to inflammation with disintegration of the follicle epithelium and destruction of the follicle structures.

Analogously, cytotoxic alterations between lymphocytes and beta cells as well as beta cell degeneration in the course of insulitis point to an autoimmune mechanism at the level of the pancreatic islets. Furthermore, cellular decay is evidenced by the demonstration of phagocytosed cell debris in macrophages. Islet fibrosis as observed in cattle after prolonged immunization (Le Compte et al., 1966) can at last be considered a final state of this autoaggressive immune mechanism. Whether the secretory hypertrophy of the still intact beta cells also represents an early cytotoxic alteration seems doubtful. Perhaps these changes may rather be interpreted as an attempt to compensate an insulin deficiency due to the progressive destruction of beta cells.

Since lymphocytic insulitis develops after immunization with insulin, its inducing factor has to be sought in the antigenicity of crystalline insulin. The antigenicity of diverse insulins could be demonstrated in many species (MOLONEY and COVAL, 1955; MOLONEY and APRILE, 1959; ARQUILLA and FINN, 1963; HIRATA and BLUMENTHAL, 1963; BRUNFELDT and DECKERT, 1964). The antibodies thus formed have been identified as immunoglobulins of IgG, IgM, IgA and IgE type (YAGI *et al.*, 1963; HORINO *et al.*, 1966; DOLOVICH *et al.*, 1970).

In addition to the production of humoral antibodies, immunization with insulin evokes a cellular immune response characterizing delayed hypersensitivity (RENOLD *et al.*, 1969; FEDERLIN *et al.*, 1968; FEDERLIN, 1971). Furthermore, several studies have revealed that not only heterologous but also homologous insulins act as antigens. In cattle (RENOLD *et al.*, 1964, 1966), sheep (RENOLD *et al.*, 1969), pigs (BRUNFELDT and DECKERT, 1964) rabbits (FELLENBERG and ROSE, 1968) and guinea pigs (FENTON *et al.*, 1963; GUTSCHMIDT, 1973) circulating antibodies against injected homologous insulin could be demonstrated.

This phenomenon may primarily be explained in terms of molecular changes which occur during the extraction of insulin, thereby producing antigenicity. Studies by BERSON and YALOW (1961, 1963) and LOCKWOOD and PROUT (1962) indicate that differences in the tertiary structure between endogenous, circulating and exogenous, extracted insulin rather than changes in the amino acid sequence may account for antigenicity. Further possibilities concerning the antigenicity of homologous insulin include the concept that endogenous insulin is associated with other plasma proteins leading to the covering or modification of an antigenic site on either molecule. Chemical procedures might result in an uncovering of the antigenic site of the insulins (RENOLD *et al.*, 1964). However, none of these theories has yet been confirmed. Regarding the studies on insulitis in immunization with homologous and heterologous insulins in rabbits and other species, it also remains unknown, wether chemical alterations of the insulins due to extraction procedures may account for the extent and the character of the immunological response. Thus, it remains open why all animals thus far examined formed humoral insulin antibodies which can be associated with delayed hypersensitivity (FEDERLIN, 1971), whereas insulitis representing an autoimmune mechanism is, in addition, found only in cattle, sheep and rabbits. For example, no histopathological islet lesions in pigs (BRUNFELDT and DECKERT, 1964) and dogs (MENZEL and ZIEGLER, 1970) immunized with porcine or bovine insulin have been reported. Guinea pigs generally lack typical insulitis when immunized either with heterologous (FEDERLIN, 1971; FREYTAG, 1972) or homologous insulin (GUTSCHMIDT, 1973), although, in addition to the production of circulating antibodies (HIRATA and BLUMENTHAL, 1963; FENTON *et al.*, 1963), delayed hypersensitivity can be demonstrated (FEDERLIN, 1971). Single observations of lymphocytic infiltrates at the level of the pancreatic islets in guinea pigs (FREYTAG, 1972; FEDERLIN, 1971) are probably exceptional findings. Rabbits showing marked insulitis after immunization with bovine insulin develop no insulitis when immunized with porcine (Klöppel et al., 1972) or rabbit insulin (Fellenberg and Rose, 1968). Lastly, it should be mentioned that islet infiltrates have also never been observed in diabetics treated with insulin.

The different immunological behavior of the single species with regard to immunization with insulin may possibly also be caused by the variable parallelism in amino acid sequence of the insulins. On the basis of this theory it may be suggested that a strong parallelism in primary structure leads to only poor formation of circulating antibodies on one hand, but to insulitis on the other. Thus, the far-reaching identity in the amino acid sequences of porcine and rabbit insulin would, for example, account for the low level of antibody production in rabbits immunized with porcine insulin. Moreover, the well-known property of guinea pigs to form large amounts of antibodies to beef or porcine insulin would be explained by the great differences in primary structure between guinea pig insulin and bovine or porcine insulin. As for insulitis, however, the theory fails to make the species-specific occurrence of this islet lesion conceivable. The findings mentioned above show that immunization with homologous insulin—an insulin with an identical amino acid sequence—will obviously evoke lymphocytic islet infiltration in only in a few species while many others lack it. Furthermore, despite the close relationship in primary structure between porcine and rabbit insulin, i.e., the two insulins are identical at 50 out of 51 positions, no insulitis is found in rabbits injected with porcine insulin. On the other hand, the administration of bovine insulin, which differs at 3 out of 51 positions, elicits insulitis in the same species. In summary, in connection with many studies concerning the mode of antigenicity of insulins (for references see Pfeiffer et al., 1969) these findings show that identity or difference in amino acid sequence of various insulins may only slightly account for the differences in their immunological behavior.

The recent discovery of proinsulin, the single polypeptide chain precursor of insulin, by Steiner and associates (Steiner et al., 1968) presented new possibilities for explaining the antigenicity of the crystalline insulin preparations. The detailed analysis of the amino acid sequence of porcine (Chance et al., 1968) and bovine proinsulin (Steiner et al., 1970) revealed that their connecting peptide sequences differ at 17 out of 33 positions whereas the insulins themselves differ only at 2 out of 51 positions. These structural variations are reflected in the high degree of immunological specifity shown by these proteins when tested with various proinsulin antisera (Rubenstein et al., 1970). Furthermore, small amounts (usually less than two percent) of proinsulin and intermediate forms were detected in crystalline insulin preparations by gel filtration (Steiner et al., 1968). According to the studies of Schlichtkrull (1970) on crystalline porcine insulin, the "crude" proinsulin fractions (dimer insulin, proinsulin, intermediate forms and as yet uncharacterized proteins) are very good antigens whose antibodies strongly cross react with the so-called "monocomponent" insulin fraction and neutralize its biological effect to some extent. Monocomponent porcine insulin injected in rabbits evokes, on the other hand, no antibody production. From this point of view it is therefore impossible to define exactly the antigen eliciting insulitis when normal crystalline insulin is injected. But in terms of the destruction of the normal islet architecture and the disappearance of beta cells in experimental insulitis, one can suggest that the insulitis antigen, though it is possibly not identical with the pure monocomponent insulin, probably belongs to the insulin-related proteins.

RENOLD et al. (1968) as well as LEE et al. (1969) pointed out that the highest titer of circulating antibodies to insulin was observed in animals with the most marked insulitis. Accordingly, an association between humoral and cellular immune mechanisms seems to exist. Our own studies, however, are not in accordance with this concept since there was no significant relation between the level of the antibody titer and the severeness of the insulitis. As mentioned above, the rabbit showing the highest antibody titer had no insulitis, while the rabbit with the most striking islet infiltrates exhibited a very low insulin-binding capacity of the serum. In opposition to the observations cited above these results may reflect that experimental insulitis in rabbits immunized with insulin can develop without relation to the degree of humoral antibody production. Findings of TORESON et al. (1968) may also be interpreted in the same way. They observed the first cellular infiltrates in the pancreas of rabbits before immunoreactive antibodies could be demonstrated. A lack of dependence between the titer of antibody and the severeness of the histopathological lesion has also been reported in experimental orchitis (RÜMKE, 1969).

Of the species immunized with insulin, only rabbits showed transient hyperglycemia or even frank diabetes, in a small number of instances (TORESON et al., 1968; LEE et al., 1969; KLÖPPEL et al., 1972). Since the occurrence of a decreased tolerance to glucose correlates better in time with the development of insulitis than with the periods of maximum circulating antibody, the islet lesion is considered as an inducing factor of decreased tolerance to glucose (LEE et al., 1969). On the basis of the findings in cattle (RENOLD et al., 1966), sheep (RENOLD et al., 1969) and rabbits (KLÖPPEL et al., 1972), however, no clear evidence is provided that hyperglycemia is caused by an immune-pathological lesion at the level of the pancreatic islets. Despite progressive islet changes in cows and sheep during a prolonged immunization period, decreased tolerance to glucose could never be guaranteed. Furthermore, transient hyperglycemia of up to 280 mg/100 ml was also observed in rabbits immunized with porcine insulin. Moreover, hyperglycemic episodes also appeared in rabbits immunized with bovine insulin but which did not have insulitis. In contrast, a correlation existed between an elevation in blood glucose and the level of antibody titer. Thus, rabbits with transient hyperglycemia exhibited on the average higher antibody titers than monoglycemic animals. This correlation was independent of the existence or the severeness of an insulitis. On the basis of these data it seems likely that the diabetic state in these animals is due to biological neutralization of endogenous insulin by its binding to circulating antibodies. This was evidenced by Grodsky (1965) who showed that insulin antibodies in man and rabbits not only react with exogenous but also with endogenous insulin. The paradoxical reaction of blood sugar in some immunized guinea pigs a short time after the injection of insulin without adjuvant points also to a temporary neutralization of endogenous insulin activity by stimulated antibodies (Freytag and Menke, 1970).

V. Summary and Conclusions

In summarizing the findings and concepts concerning experimental insulitis in some species immunized with insulin, it can be stated that the lymphocytic infiltrate of the pancreatic islets probably represents a cellular immune response with autoimmune character. Since this form of an experimental insulitis closely resembles the inflammatory islet lesions in juvenile diabetics, immuno-pathological mechanisms are also discussed in the pathogenesis and etiology of insulitis in man. However, despite important experimental hypotheses of the immunological genesis of insulitis, no clear evidence is yet available that diabetes in man may indeed be caused by immune mechanisms directed against insulin or other components of the endocrine pancreas.

E. Experimental Insulitis in Animals Injected with Anti-Insulin Serum

The possible significance of immunopathologic mechanisms for the pathogenesis of insulitis in newborns of diabetic mothers may be supported by findings on the pancreatic islets in animals injected with anti-insulin serum of guinea pigs. After treatment with insulin antibodies animals show a polymorphocellular inflammation within the pancreas, involving only the islet tissue. Small rodents such as mice and rats are most suitable for developing insulitis since only small amounts of anti-insulin serum are required to produce insular inflammation in these animals.

I. Specific Properties of Guinea Pig Anti-Insulin Serum

In order to evoke insulitis under the experimental conditions of passive immunization it is necessary to use anti-insulin serum from guinea pigs because of the special characteristics of the antibodies to insulin in these species. As shown previously by Moloney and Coval (1955) and Moloney and Goldsmith (1957), only the insulin antibodies of guinea pigs were able to induce hyperglycemia in a number of experimental animals (Armin et al., 1961). Later, this was confirmed by many authors, who demonstrated a strong neutralizing effect of guinea pig antibodies on the biological activity of endogenously secreted insulin by immunological binding to the hormone (WRIGHT *et al.*, 1962; ARQUILLA *et al.*, 1962; CUNNINGHAM *et al.*, 1963; ARQUILLA *et al.*, 1966). A further characteristic and important property of guinea pig anti-insulin serum is that it contains rather constantly high amounts of precipi-tating antibodies to insulin (JONES and CUNLIFE, 1961).

II. History

LACY *et al.* (1963) and LACY and WRIGHT (1965) were the first to find an infiltrate consisting predominantly of eosinophilic leukocytes in the pan-creatic tissue 4 to 31 hours after intraperitoneal injection of anti-insulin serum from guinea pig. In particular, they observed a diffuse pancreatic edema and focal necrosis or hemorrhage of the acinar tissue. In contrast the islets appear-ed normal except for the degranulated beta cells. The infiltration of eosino-philes only involved the islets when the antiserum was injected intravenously. The authors suggested that these findings are based on immunological mecha-nisms at the pancreatic level. They therefore described the lesions as "allergic interstitial pancreatitis". Similar studies were performed by LOGOTHETOPOULOS and BELL (1966). In order to study the regeneration of beta cells during prolonged hyperglycemia mice were injected intraperitoneally with the glo-bulin fraction of anti-insulin sera so that blood glucose levels were maintained over 280 mg/100 ml. Inflammatory cells around the islets with heavily degra-nulated beta cells could be observed 24 hours after the beginning of the study, whereas the exocrine pancreatic portion was free of inflammation. The small infiltrates consisted of eosinophilic and neutrophilic granulocytes as well as of some mononuclear cells. The extent of insulitis slowly increased until the third day of the study and remained constant thereafter. During the course of the study the cytological character of the infiltrate appeared to change. Besides polymorphonuclear cells more and more mononuclear cells were present. The degranulated beta cells showed signs of marked cellular hyperactivity after prolonged treatment. The incorporation of ^{3}H-thymidine in beta cell nuclei, indicating an increase in mitotic activity, reached a peak at the third day of the study.

III. Histopathology

In our studies on insulitis in mice and rats (FREYTAG *et al.*, 1969; FREYTAG and KLÖPPEL, 1969; KLÖPPEL *et al.*, 1970; KLÖPPEL *et al.*, 1971; FREYTAG, 1972) injected intravenously with anti-insulin serum from guinea pigs, the inflammatory process develops as follows.

1. Acute Type of Insulitis

A single injection of 0.02 ml anti-insulin serum/g body weight leads to pure granulocytic infiltration around the islets, reaching its maximum after 3 to 6 hours. The extent of the infiltrates, particularly in mice, depends on the

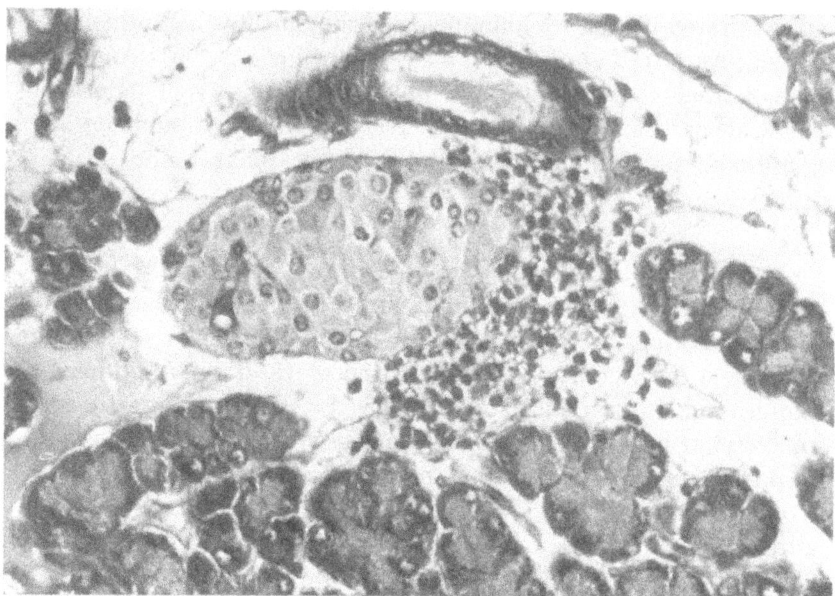

Fig. 12. Mice pancreas 180 minutes after injection of high titer anti-insulin serum. Peri-insular infiltrate of eosinophiles and neutrophiles (acute insulitis). PAS. × 300

titer of the injected anti-insulin serum. Ninety minutes after injection an intra-vascular aggregation of leukocytes can be observed in a number of instances, accompanied by perivascular edema. Only single leukocytes are emigrated. By means of tritium-labelled dextran with a definite molecular weight comparable to that of albumin, an increased permeability of islet sinusoids and the adjacent vessels can be demonstrated. Around these small veins the first extravasations are then detected. By 180 minutes after the injection, edema and granulocytic infiltrates are localized primarily in the periinsular area (Fig. 12). The dilated sinusoids within the islets frequently contained PAS-positive material having the same histologic appearance as hyaline thrombi. The islets are now clearly demarcated. By 360 minutes after the beginning of the study the infiltrates enroach on the islets, and in a number of cases small groups of granulocytes are observed around the sinusoids. The inflammation then continues for some hours. Later it decreases slowly and disappears completely after 48 hours.

In principle this acute type of insulitis follows the same course in rats and mice. However, the extent of acute insulitis in mice appears to be more dependent on the level of the antibody titer, while in rats no certain relationship between the occurrence of insulitis and the quality of injected anti-insulin serum seems to exist. Thus, the injection of low titer [insulin binding capacity (IBC): 0.2 to 1 U/ml], of medium titer (IBC 2 to 5 U/ml) and of high titer anti-insulin serum (IBC: 6 to 11 U/ml) results in different degrees of degranulation of beta cells. There are also different degrees of granulocytic infiltration and variably marked occurrence of hyaline thrombi. Differences in the histo-

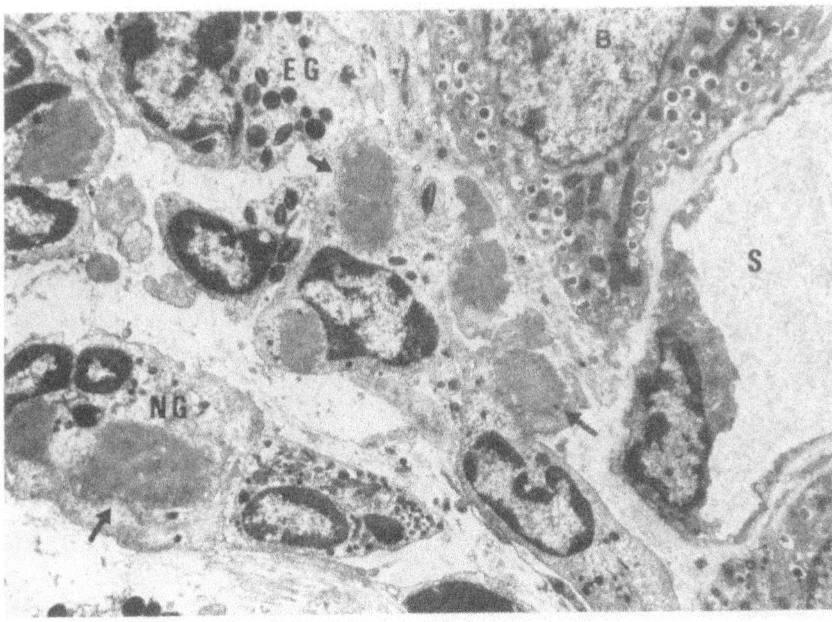

Fig. 13. Mice pancreas 180 minutes after repeated injection of high titer anti-insulin serum. Polymorphocellular insulitis within and around the islet (acute insulitis). Interstitial infiltration by eosinophilic (*EG*) and neutrophilic granulocytes (*NG*). Precipitated material in close contact to a beta cell (*B*) being phagocytosed by neutrophiles (↑). Sinusoid (*S*). × 9700. (From KLÖPPEL *et al.*, 1971 b)

logical appearance of the islet lesions also seem to exist when mice are treated either with antiserum to porcine insulin or with antiserum to bovine insulin, both having similar insulin binding capacities. Too much emphasis, however, should not be placed on these findings, for there is no clear-cut distinction between the single histologic pictures in the two groups.

Electron microscopic examination of acute insulitis very often revealed cloudy electron dense material within the sinusoids 90 minutes after single injection of anti-insulin serum. In addition the micrographs confirm the aggregation of eosinophilic and neutrophilic granulocytes within and partly around the small islet vessels. After 180 minutes the emigration of eosinophiles and neutrophiles is fully developed (Fig. 13). Furthermore, cloudy electron dense material, probably representing precipitated insulin-antibody complexes, is found in the vicinity of beta cells already being phagocytosed by neutrophilic granulocytes.

In consequence of the diabetic syndrome, induced by strong neutralization of biologic activity of insulin, hyperactivity of beta cells will be observed (LOGOTHETOPOULOS, 1968; KLÖPPEL *et al.*, 1971). Within a few hours following a single injection, a heavy degranulation occurs with displacement of the remaining granules to the cell surface. In addition there is an enlargement of the Golgi complexes and an increased number of microvesicles and pregranules, representing immature granules. In an extreme state of functional overstrain

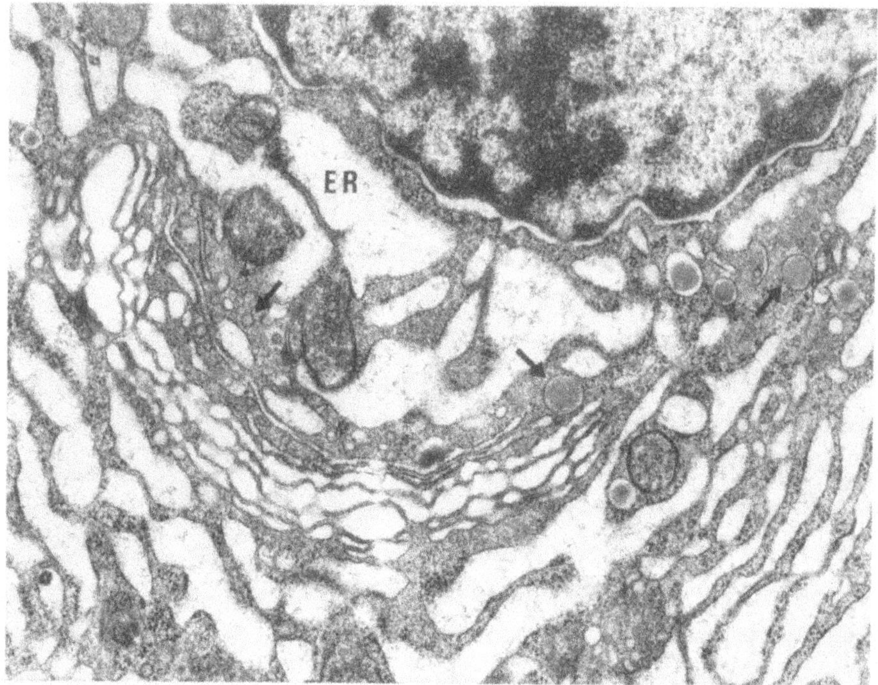

Fig. 14. Mice pancreas 360 minutes after injection of high titer anti-insulin serum. Hypersecretory degeneration of a beta cell with cystical transformation of the rough endoplasmic reticulum, shrinkage of the nucleus and heavy degranulation. In the vicinity of the enlarged Golgi complex microvesicles and pregranules (↑). × 22100. (From Klöppel *et al.*, 1971 b)

sometimes a hypersecretory degeneration of beta cells is observed characterized by shrinkage of the nucleus and cystic deformation of the rough endoplasmic reticulum (Fig. 14).

2. Chronic Types of Insulitis

Continuation of the injections (0.02 to 0.04 ml/g body weight daily) generally results in the continuing polymorphocellular inflammation of islets, in an increased occurrence of hyaline thrombi within the islets and in islet hyperplasia. Depending on the level of insulin antibody titer, the dosage, the injection of anti-bovine or anti-porcine insulin serum or the globulin fraction of these sera, a subacute, chronic recurrent and chronic insulitis can be distinguished. The extent of the infiltrate and the deposition of PAS-positive material in the sinusoids depend in principle on the level of the antibody titer. The administration of high and medium titer antisera evokes a marked islet decomposition by peri- and intrainsular insulitis (Fig. 15), leads to the development of large hyaline thrombi (Fig. 16), and sometimes causes focal necrosis within the islets (subacute and chronic recurrent insulitis). As in acute insulitis

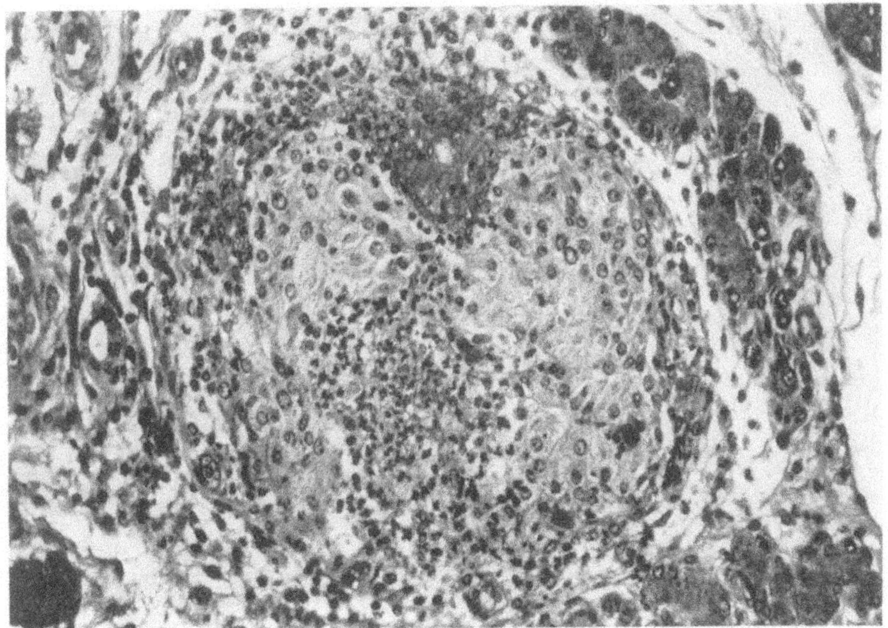

Fig. 15. Mice pancreas 3 days after repeated injections of high titer anti-insulin serum. Polymorphocellular insulitis within and around the islet (subacute insulitis). PAS. × 300

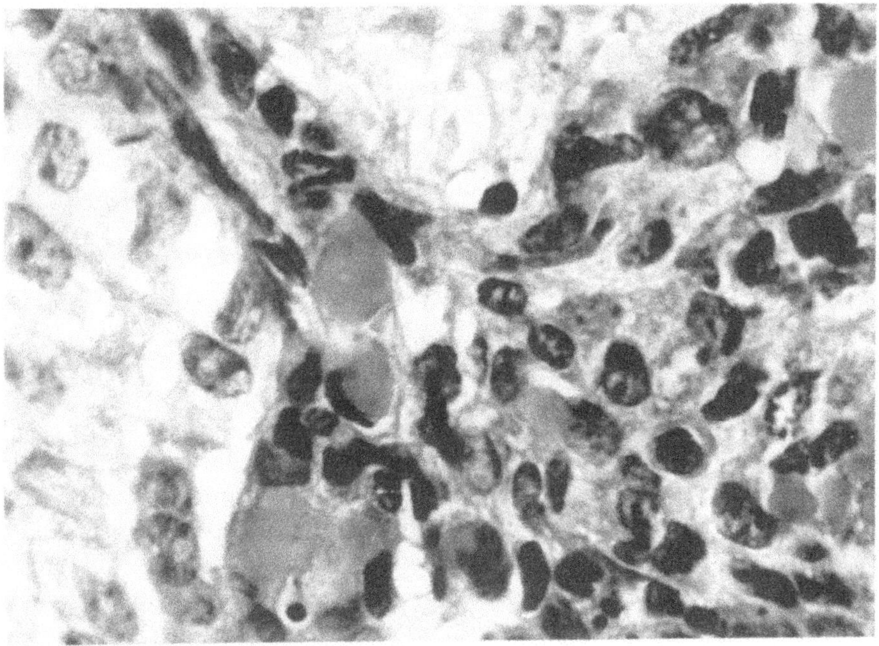

Fig. 16. Mice pancreas after repeated injections of anti-insulin serum. Large hyaline thrombi in the dilated sinusoids associated with polymorphocellular infiltration (chronic recurrent insulitis). PAS. × 1200

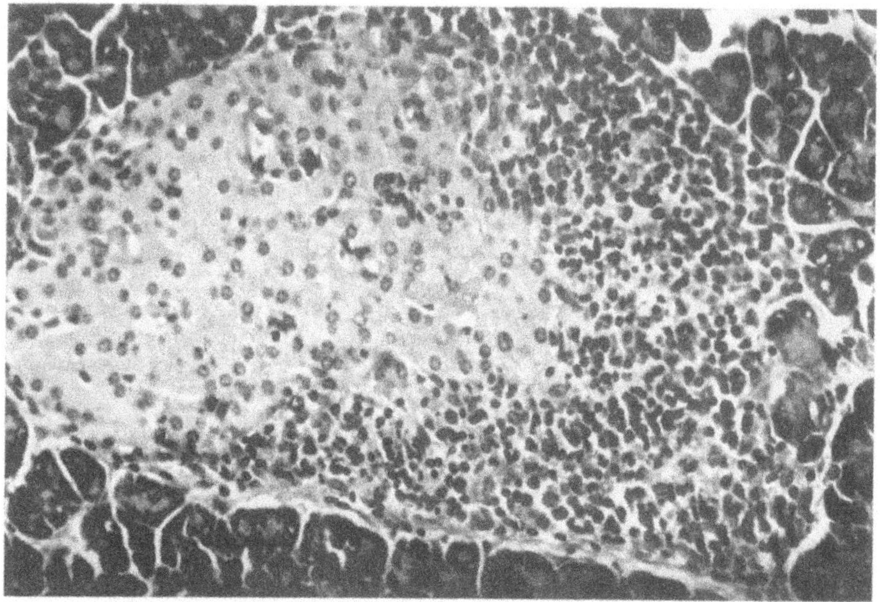

Fig. 17. Mice pancreas after repeated injections of medium titer anti-insulin serum over 6 weeks. Half-moon like infiltrate consisting mainly of mononucleated cells (chronic insulitis). PAS. × 300

the islets in chronic recurrent insulitis appear to contain more hyaline thrombi and less inflammatory cells when anti-porcine insulin instead of anti-bovine insulin serum is injected. The cytological composition of the infiltrate remains almost unchanged in these cases. However, when smaller dosages are administered, antisera of medium or low capacity are used, or when only the globulin fraction is injected, the cytological character of the infiltrate will change. The granulocytes, prevalent in the beginning, are increasingly displaced by mononuclear cells. Moreover, only scattered hyaline thrombi are observed. Occasionally development of the infiltration, consisting mainly of round mononucleated cells, runs a typical course in chronic insulitis. The infiltration starts in the vicinity of a small vein adjacent to an islet, and progressively extends towards the peri-insular space. The proliferation of large round cells finally results in the formation of a half-moon like infiltrate around the islets, accompanied by pericapillary formation of collagen within the islets (Fig. 17). In long term studies of up to six weeks the infiltrates sometimes encroach along the vessels upon the islets, destroying the normal islet architecture.

When the administration of anti-insulin serum is stopped, the islet changes usually recede within one week. At the same time occurrence of fibrocytes within and around the islets, associated with islet fibrosis, is obvious in cases of chronic recurrent and chronic insulitis. Persistent infiltrates are only rarely found. Nevertheless, some of the animals show a slightly decreased tolerance to glucose even though treatment has been discontinued. Electron micrographs of chronic insulitis show that the infiltrate consists of immunoblasts,

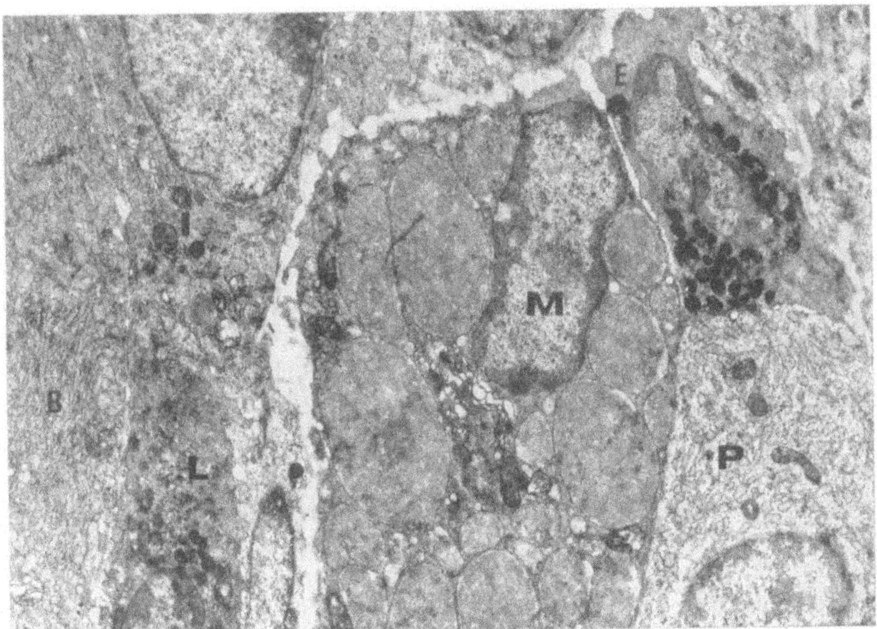

Fig. 18. Mice pancreas after repeated injections of high titer anti-insulin serum. Part of the polymorphocellular infiltrate within an islet: macrophage (*M*), containing phago-cytosed material, lymphocyte of the intermediate type (*L*), immunoblast (*I*), eosiniphilic granulocyte (*E*), plasma cell (*P*), beta cell (*B*). × 5400. (From KLÖPPEL *et al.*, 1972)

frequently acting as macrophages, some lymphocytes and few plasma cells (Fig. 18). Furthermore, large amounts of cloudy electron dense material are observed, localized mainly in the extracellular space adjacent to beta cells, where it is phagocytosed by macrophages.

Pronounced hyperactivity of beta cells is obvious as long as the diabetic syndrome continues. The beta cell in particular displays hyperplasia of the rough endoplasmic reticulum, associated with heavy degranulation and fre-quent immaturity of the remaining granules. The expansion of the endoplasmic reticulum can proceed, resulting in cystic transformation. In association with shrinkage of nucleus and scattered granules within the cytoplasm, this altera-tion characterizes hypersecretory degeneration. The signs of hyperactivity disappear when the diabetic syndrome vanishes.

IV. Pathogenesis and Etiology

Single and repeated injections of guinea pig anti-insulin serum result in temporary hyperglycemia, accompanied morphologically by the development of polymorphocellular insulitis and hyperactivity of the beta cells. The pres-ence of cloudy electron dense material within the islet sinusoids within 90 minutes after serum injection indicates that newly secreted insulin is precipi-tated by the antibody in the islet area. Adequate precipitates are lacking in other organs. The electron dense material is therefore thought to be the precipitated complexes of insulin with its antibody. At the light microscopic level evidence for the immunological origin of the hyaline thrombi in the islet sinusoids is provided by the specific fluorescence of this material after injection of anti-insulin serum containing fluorescein isothiocyanate-labelled insulin antibodies. As is known from the phenomenon of Arthus, the production of antigen-antibody complexes results in activation of the complement system, which initiates a leukotactic process. The aggregated eosinophilic and neutrophilic granulocytes release mediators, leading to permeability and dilatation of the small veins. Morphologically, an analogous process, which depends in its degree on the level of the anti-insulin serum titer, starts in the area of the pancreatic islets. This also suggests that acute insulitis following the injection of anti-insulin serum represents an immune reaction of the immediate type, comparable with local Arthus phenomenon.

The precipitated immune complexes are initially phagocytosed by leukocytes. Later they are found in macrophages which become preponderant in the infiltrate. In addition to these cells small lymphocytes and lymphocytes of the intermediate type are obvious. Also single plasma cells are seen. Since these cells are usually associated with a cellular immune response of the delayed type, it is likely that in long-term studies the immune reaction of the immediate type is more and more superposed by an immune response of the delayed type, possibly induced by the precipitated immunoglobulins of guinea pigs. Uhr et al. (1957) showed that injection of small amounts of antigen-antibody complexes, made with an excess of antibody, are able to evoke cellular hypersensitivity. Similar conditions are also provided in the insulitis model under discussion.

It remains unclear why repeated injections of the globulin fraction or of anti-insulin serum in a small dosage and with low titers sometimes result in chronic insulitis, characterized from the beginning by its mononucleated cells. Possibly the amounts of the antibodies play a role in the cytological differentiation of this infiltrate, although there is no clear-cut correlation between these two factors. Furthermore, it is an open question why animals show differences in the patterns of insulitis when injected either with anti-bovine or anti-porcine insulin antibodies. These findings may indicate that guinea pigs immunized with bovine insulin produce in part different types of antibodies with binding sites other than those produced by guinea pigs treated with porcine insulin. However, it is totally unknown whether there are really different types of antibodies to porcine and bovine insulin.

V. Summary and Conclusions

Insulitis in mice and rats injected with anti-insulin serum from guinea pigs is thought to be an immune reaction, and may be compared with a local Arthus phenomenon. The infiltrate, consisting of eosinophiles and neutrophiles, and the demonstration of precipitated material in the islet area suggest an immune response of the immediate type. The occurrence of mononuclear cells in the long-term studies indicates that delayed hypersensitivity against foreign immunoglobulins in the insulin-antibody complexes may also develop. Since patterns of chronic polymorphocellular insulitis correspond well with histological findings in the pancreas of newborns of diabetic mothers, immunological factors could also be responsible for these findings in man. Insulitis in juvenile diabetics, on the other hand, can hardly be interpreted by the histopathologic results in the experimental insulitis under discussion.

References

ARMIN, J., CUNNINGMAN, N. F., GRANT, R. T., LLOYD, M. K., WRIGHT, P. H.: Acute insulin deficiency provoked in the dog, pig, and sheep by single injection of anti-insulin serum. J. Physiol. (Lond.) 157, 64 (1961).

ARQUILLA, E. R., ALEXANDER, J., PTACEK, E., LOOSLI, E.: Studies on insulin neutralization by antisera from various species. I. Methodology and assay of insulin with intact anesthetized rats. Diabetes 11, 412 (1962).

ARQUILLA, E. R., FINN, J.: Insulin antibody variations in rabbits and guinea pigs and multiple antigenetic determinants on insulin. J. exp. Med. 118, 55 (1963).

ARQUILLA, E. R., OOMS, H., FINN, J.: Genetic differences of combining sites of insulin antibodies and importance of C-terminal portion of the A chain to biological and immunological activity of insulin. Diabetologia 2, 1 (1966).

ASSCHE, F. A. van: A morphological study of the Langerhans' islets of the fetal pancreas in late pregnancy. Biol. Neonat. (Basel) 14, 19 (1968).

ASSCHE, F. A. van: The fetal endocrine pancreas. A quantitative morphological approach. Proefschrift ingediend bij de faculteit Geneeskunde der Katholieke Universiteit Leuven, 1970.

BAIRD, J. D., FARQUHAR, J. W.: The insulin secreting capacity of the pancreas in the newborn infants of normal and diabetic women. Lancet 1962 I, 71.

BARBIERI, V.: Pancreatit. Subac. e glicosur. Secund. etc. Gazz. Osp. Clin. 30, 273 (1909).

BARBONI, E., MANOCCHIO, I.: Alterazioni pancreatiche in bovinicon diabete mellito post-aftoso. Arch. vet. ital. 13, 477 (1962).

BEAVEN, D. W., NELSON, D. H., RENOLD, A. E., THORN, G. W.: Diabetes mellitus and Addison's disease. New Engl. J. Med. 261, 443 (1959).

BEEK, C. van: Kan men aan een doodgeborene de diagnose diabetes mellitus der moeder stellen? Ned. T. Geneesk. 83, 5973 (1939).

BERSON, S. A., YALOW, R. S.: Immunochemical distinction between insulin with identical amino-acid sequences. Nature (Lond.) 191, 1392 (1961).

BORCHARD, F., MÜNTEFERING, H.: Beitrag zur quantitativen Morphologie der Langerhansschen Inseln bei Früh- und Neugeborenen. Virchows Arch. Abt. A 346, 178 (1969).

BROWN, E. E.: Infectious origin of juvenile diabetes. Arch. Pediat. 73, 191 (1956).

BRUNFELDT, K., DECKERT, T.: Antibodies in the pig against pig insulin. Acta endocr. (Kbh.) 47, 367 (1964).

CARDELL, B. S.: Hypertrophy and hyperplasia of the pancreatic islets in the newborn infants. J. Path. Bact. 66, 335 (1953).

CARPENTER, C. C. J., SOLOMON, N., SILVERBERG, S. G., BLEDSOE, N., NORTHCUTT, R. C., KLINGENBERG, J. R., BENNET, I. L., HARVEY, A.: Schmidt's syndrome (thyroid and adrenal insufficiency): a review of the literature and a report of 15 new cases including ten instances of coexisting diabetes mellitus. Medicine (Baltimore) 43, 153 (1964).

CECIIL, R. L.: A study of the pathological anatomy of the pancreas in 90 cases of diabetes mellitus. J. exp. Med. 11, 266 (1909).

CHANCE, R. E., ELLIS, R. M., BROMER, W. W.: Porcine proinsulin: characterization and amino acid sequence. Science 161, 165 (1968).

Chetty, M. P., Watson, K. C.: Antibody-like activity in diabetic and normal serum, measured by complement consumption. Lancet **1965** I, 947.

Cochran, C. G., Dixon, F. J.: Cell and tissue damage through antigen-antibody complexes. In: Textbook of immunopathology, ed. by P. A. Miescher and H. J. Muller-Eberhard, vol. I, p. 94–110. New York and London: Grune and Stratton 1968.

Colover, J., Glynn, L. E.: Experimental isoimmune adrenalitis. Immunology **2**, 172 (1958).

Craighead, J. E., Steinke, J.: Diabetes mellitus-like syndrome in mice infected with encephalomyocarditis virus. Amer. J. Path. **63**, 119 (1971).

Creutzfeldt, W., Theodossiou, A.: Die Relation der A- und B-Zellen in den Pankreasinseln bei Nichtdiabetikern und Diabetikern. Beitr. path. Anat. **117**, 235 (1957).

Cunningham, N. F., Patterson, D. S. P., Wright, P. H.: Acute insulin deficiency provoked in sheep and cows by single injections of anti-insulin serum. J. Physiol. (Lond.) **169**, 137 (1963).

D'Agostino, A. N., Bahn, R. C.: A histopathologic study of the pancreas of infants of diabetic mothers. Diabetes **12**, 327 (1963).

Davies, J., Lacy, P. E.: Observations on the failure of insulin to pass from the fetus to the mother in the rabbit. Amer. J. Obstet. Gynec. **74**, 514 (1957).

Dolovich, J., Schnatz, J. D., Reisman, R. E., Yagi, Y., Arbesman, C. E.: Insulin allergy and insulin resistance. Case report with immunologic studies. J. Allergy **46**, 127 (1970).

Driscoll, S. G., Benirschke, K., Curtis, G. W.: Neonatal deaths among infants of diabetic mothers. Postmortem findings in ninety-five infants. Amer. J. Dis. Child. **100**, 818 (1960).

Dubreuil, G., Anderoidas, J.: Ilots de Langerhans géants chez un nouveau-né issu de mère glucosurique. C. R. Soc. Biol. (Paris) **23**, 1491 (1920).

Farrell, H. W., Hand, A. M., Newcomb, A. L.: Infantile diabetes. Diabetes **2**, 85 (1953).

Federlin, K.: Immunopathology of insulin. Clinical and experimental studies. Monographs on endocrinology, vol. 6, edit. by F. Gross, A. Labhart, T. Mann, L. T. Samuels and J. Zander. Berlin–Heidelberg–New York: Springer 1971.

Federlin, K., Renold, A. E., Pfeiffer, E. F.: Antigenbinding leucocytes in patients and in insulinsensitized animals with delayed insulin allergy. Immunopathology, Vth Int. Symposion, ed. by P. A. Miescher and P. Grabar, p. 107 Basel–Stuttgart: Schwabe & Co. Publ. 1968.

Fellenberg, v. R., Rose, N. R.: Antigenicity of insulin. Int. Arch. Allergy **33**, 454 (1968).

Fenton, E. L., Mann, C. B., Pope, C. G., Smith, G. H.: The production of circulating autoantibodies to guinea pig insulin. Abstr. Progr. Autumn Meeting of Med. Scient. Sect. of Brit. Diabet. Ass. 1963.

Ferner, H.: Das Inselsystem des Pankreas. Stuttgart: Georg Thieme 1952.

Fischer, B.: Pankreas und Diabetes. Frankfurt. Z. Path. **17**, 218 (1915).

Freytag, G.: Histologische und autoradiographische Untersuchungen am Inselsystem der Maus beim Insulinantikörper-Diabetes. Beitr. path. Anat. **137**, 121 (1968).

Freytag, G.: Immunpathologie des Diabetes mellitus. Veröffentlichungen aus der Morphologischen Pathologie, vol. 88, edit. by W. Giese, W. Büngler, G. Seifert und G. Peters. Stuttgart: Gustav Fischer 1972.

Freytag, G.: Do virus serve as mediators of immunologic reactions? Franc qui Foundation Colloquium, 1973 (in press).

Freytag, G., Klöppel, G.: Experimentelle Insulitis und Pankreatitis nach Immunseren gegen Pankreasextrakte verschiedener Reinheitsgrade. Beitr. path. Anat. **39**, 138 (1969).

Freytag, G., Klöppel, G., Howe, I.: Zur Pathogenese der experimentellen Insulitis. Verh. dtsch. Ges. Path. **53**, 423 (1969).

Freytag, G., Menke, B.: Latenter Diabetes mellitus bei Meerschweinchen während der aktiven Immunisierung gegen Fremdinsulin. 16. Symp. Dtsch. Ges. Endokrinologie, p. 65. Berlin—Heidelberg—New York: Springer 1970.

Gamble, D. R., Kinsley, M. L., Fitzgerald, M. G., Bolton, R., Taylor, K. W.: Viral antibodies in diabetes mellitus. Brit. J. Med. **3**, 627 (1969).

Gepts, W.: Contribution á l'étude morphologique des îslots de Langerhans au cours du diabète. Ann. Soc. roy. Sci. méd. nat. Brux. **10**, 5 (1957).

GEPTS, W.: Pathologic anatomy of the pancreas in juvenile diabetes mellitus. Diabetes **14**, 619 (1965).

GRODSKY, G. M.: Production of autoantibodies to insulin in man and rabbit. Diabetes **14**, 396 (1965).

GRODSKY, G. M., FELDMAN, R., TORESON, W. E., LEE, J. C.: Diabetes mellitus in rabbits immunized with insulin. Diabetes **15**, 579 (1966).

GUNDERSEN, E.: Is diabetes of infectious origin? J. infect. Dis. **41**, 197 (1927).

GUTSCHMIDT, G.: Immunologische und morphologische Befunde nach aktiver Immunisierung von Meerschweinchen gegen homologes Insulin. Dissertation. Universität Hamburg 1973.

HEIBERG, K. A.: Ein interessanter Fall zur Beleuchtung der Pathogenese und der pathologischen Anatomie des Diabetes mellitus. Zbl. ges. Physiol. u. Path. des Stoffwechsels **5**, 609 (1910).

HEIBERG, K. A.: Über Diabetes bei Kindern. Arch. Kinderheilk. **56**, 403 (1911).

HELWIG, E. B.: Hypertrophy and hyperplasia of islands of Langerhans in infants born of diabetic mothers. Arch. intern. Med. **65**, 221 (1940).

HIRATA, Y., BLUMENTHAL, H. T.: Demonstration of a precipitating insulin-binding antibody in the sera of insulin treated guinea pigs and rabbits. J. Lab. clin. Med. **62**, 683 (1963).

HORINO, M., YU, S. Y., BLUMENTHAL, H. T.: Studies on experimental insulin immunity. I. Dynamics of insulin immunity in the guinea pig. Diabetes **15**, 812 (1966).

HULTQUIST, G., DAHLEN, M., HELANDER, C. G.: Über die Technik bei Darstellung und Zählung der sog. Silberzellen in den Langerhans'schen Inseln. Schweiz. Z. Path. **11**, 570 (1948).

IRVINE, W. J., CLARKE, B. F., SCARTH, L., CULLEN, D. R., DUNCAN, L. J. P.: Thyroid and gastric autoimmunity in patients with diabetes mellitus. Lancet **1970I**, 163.

JANKOVIC, B. D., ISVANESKI, M., POPESKOVIC, L., MITROVIC, K.: Experimental allergic thyroiditis (and parathyroiditis) in neonatally thymectomized and bursectomized chickens. Participation of the thymus in the development of disease. Int. Arch. Allergy **26**, 18 (1965).

JOHN, H. J.: Diabetes mellitus in children. J. Pediat. **35**, 723 (1949).

JONES, V. E., CUNLIFFE, A. C.: Precipitating antibody to insulin. Nature (Lond.) **192**, 136 (1961).

KÅRESEN, R.: Experimental allergic thyroiditis in the guinea pig. Acta path. microbiol. scand., Sect. A **78**, 625 (1970).

KLÖPPEL, G., ALTENÄHR, E., FREYTAG, G.: Elektronenmikroskopische Untersuchungen zur experimentellen Insulitis nach Injektion von Anti-Insulin-Serum. Virchows Arch. Abt. A **354**, 324 (1971).

KLÖPPEL, G., ALTENÄHR, E., FREYTAG, G.: Studies on ultrastructure und immunology of the insulitis in rabbits immunized with insulin. Virchows Arch. Abt. A **356**, 1–15 (1972).

KLÖPPEL, G., FREYTAG, G., GUTSCHMIDT, S.: Die histologischen Veränderungen des Inselorgans der Maus nach Anti-Schweine-Insulin- und Anti-Rinder-Insulin-Serum-Injektionen in Abhängigkeit von Versuchsdauer und Titerhöhe. Acta endocr. (Kbh.), Suppl. **152**, 50 (1971).

KLÖPPEL, G., FREYTAG, G., LYHS, R.: Immunhistologische Untersuchungen zum experimentellen Immun-Diabetes. Verh. dtsch. Ges. Path. **54**, 670 (1970).

KRAUS, E. J.: Die pathologisch-anatomischen Veränderungen des Pankreas beim Diabetes mellitus. In: Handbuch der speziellen pathologischen Anatomie und Histologie, edit. by F. Henke and O. Lubarsch. vol. 5, p. 622. Berlin: Springer 1929.

KREMER, H. U.: Juvenile diabetes as a sequel to mumps. Amer. J. Med. **3**, 257 (1947).

LACY, P. E., WRIGHT, P. H.: Allergic interstitial pancreatitis in rats injected with guinea pig anti-insulin serum. Diabetes **14**, 634 (1965).

LACY, P. E., WRIGHT, P. H., SILVERMAN, J. L.: Eosinophile infiltration in the pancreas of rats injected with anti-insulin serum. Fed. Proc. **22**, 604 (1963).

LANDING, B. H., PETTIT, M. D., WIENS, R. L., KNOWLES, H., GUEST, G. M.: Antithyroid antibody and chronic thyroiditis in diabetes (Letter to the Editor) J. clin. Endocr. **23**, 119 (1963).

Le COMPTE, P. M.: "Insulitis" in early juvenile diabetes. Arch. Path. **66**, 450 (1958).

Le Compte, P. M., Steinke, J., Soeldner, J. S., Renold, A. E.: Changes in the islets of Langerhans in cows injected with heterologous and homologous insulin. Diabetes 15, 586 (1966).

Lee, J. C., Grodsky, G. M., Caplan, C. J., Craw, L.: Experimental immune diabetes in the rabbit. Amer. J. Path. 57, 597 (1969).

Lockwood, D. H., Prout, T. E.: Isoantibodies to insulin. Clin. Res. 10, 401 (1962).

Logothetopoulos, J.: Electron microscopy of the pancreatic islets stimulated by insulin antibody. Canad. J. Physiol. Pharmacol. 46, 40 (1968).

Logothetopoulos, J., Bell, E. G.: Histological and autoradiographic studies of the islets of mice injected with insulin antibody. Diabetes 15, 205 (1966).

Lupulescu, 1965.

Maclean, N., Ogilvie, R. F.: Quantitative estimation of the pancreatic islet tissue in diabetic subjects. Diabetes 8, 83 (1959).

Mancini, A. M., Costanzi, G., Zampa, G. A.: Human insulin antibodies detected by immunofluorescent technique. Lancet 1964 I, 726.

Mancini, A. M., Zampa, G. A., Vecchi, A., Costanzi, G.: Histoimmunological techniques for detecting antibodies in human sera. Lancet 1965I, 1189.

McKay, D. G., Benirschke, K., Curtis, G. W.: Infants of diabetic mothers. Histologic and histochemical observations on the pancreas. Obstet. and Gynec. 2, 133 (1953).

Melin, K., Ursing, B.: Diabetes mellitus som komplikation till parotitis epidemica. Nord. Med. 60, 1715 (1958).

Menzel, R., Ziegler, M.: Zirkulierende Insulin-Antikkörper beim Hund. Endokrinologie 56, 334 (1970).

Mering, J. von, Minkowsky, O.: Diabetes mellitus nach Pankreasextirpation. Arch. exp. Path. Pharmak. 26, 371 (1889/90).

Meyenburg, H. von: Über "Insulitis" bei Diabetes. Schweiz. med. Wschr. 70, 247 (1940).

Milcou, S. M., Pop, A., Lupulescou, A., Taga, M.: L'autoimmunisation expérimentale de la surrénale chez le lapin. Ann. Endocr. (Paris) 20, 799 (1959).

Moloney, P. J., Aprile, M. A.: "On the antigenicity of insulin: flocculation of insulin-antiinsulin". Canad. J. Biochem. 37, 793 (1959).

Moloney, P. J., Coval, M.: Antigenicity of insulin: diabetes induced by specific antibodies. Biochem. J. 59, 179 (1955).

Moloney, P. J., Goldsmith, L.: On the antigenicity of insulin. Canad. J. Biochem. 35, 79 (1957).

Moore, J., Neilson, J. McE.: Gastric antibodies in diabetes mellitus. Lancet 1963II, 645.

Müntefering, H., Schmidt, W. A. K., Körber, W.: Zur Virusgenese des Diabetes mellitus bei der weißen Maus. Dtsch. med. Wschr. 96, 693 (1971).

Nagler, W., Taylor, H.: Diabetic coma with acute inflammation of islets of Langerhans. Amer. med. Ass. 184, 723 (1963).

Nerup, J., Andersen, O. O., Bendixen, G., Egeberg, J., Poulsen, J. E.: Antipancreatic cellular hypersensitivity in diabetes mellitus. Diabetes 20, 424 (1971).

Opie, E. L.: On the relation of chronic interstitial pancreatitis to the islands of Langerhans and to diabetes mellitus. J. exp. Med. 5, 393 (1901).

Opie, E. L.: Diseases of the pancreas, II. edit. Philadelphia and London 1910.

Pappenheimer, A. M., Kunz, L. J., Richardson, S.: Passage of coxsackie virus (Connecticut-5 strain) in adult mice with production of pancreatic disease. J. exp. Med. 94, 45 (1951).

Páv, J., Jezkova, Z., Skrha, F.: Insulin antibodies. Lancet 1963II, 221.

Pedersen, J.: Diabetes and pregnancy. Blood sugar of newborn infants. Copenhagen: Danish Science Press 1952 (Thesis).

Penchev, I., Andreev, D., Ditzov, S.: Insulin-precipitating antibodies in insulin treated and untreated diabetic patients. Diabetologia 4, 164 (1968).

Pfeiffer, E. F., Ditschuneit, H., Federlin, K.: Die Inselzellhormone: Die Immunologie des Insulins. In: Handbuch des Diabetes mellitus. ed. by E. F. Pfeiffer, vol. I, p. 155–201. München: J. F. Lehmann 1969.

Renold, A. E., Gonet, A. E., Vecchio, D.: Immunopathology of the endocrine pancreas. In: Textbook of immunopathology, ed. by P. A. Miescher and H. J. Müller-Eberhard, vol. II, p. 595. New York and London: Grune and Stratton 1969.

RENOLD, A. E., SOELDNER, J. S., STEINKE, J.: Immunological studies with homologous and heterologous pancreatic insulin in the cow. Ciba Found. Coll. Endocrinol. 15, 122 (1964)

RENOLD, A. E., STEINKE, J., SOELDNER, J. S., ANTONIADES, H. N., SMITL, R. E.: Immunological response to the prolanged administration of heterologous and homologous insulin in cattle. J. clin. Invest. 45, 702 (2966).

ROBINSON, B. H. B., WRIGHT, P. H.: Guinea pig anti-insulin serum. J. clin. Physiol. 155, 302 (1961).

ROY, C. C., SHAPCOTT, D. J., O'BRIEN, D.: The case for an "abnormal" insulin in diabetes mellitus. Diabetologia 4, 111 (1968).

RUBENSTEIN, A., WELBOURNE, W. P., MAKO, M., MELANI, F., STEINER, D. F.: Comparative immunology of bovine, porcine and human proinsulins and C-peptides. Diabetes 19, 546 (1970).

RÜMKE, Ph.: Antigenicity of spermatozoa. In: Textbook of immunopathology, ed. by P. A. Miescher and H. J. Müller-Eberhard, vol. II, p. 665. New York and London: Grune and Stratton 1969.

SAUERBECK, E.: Die Langerhansschen Inseln und ihre Beziehung zum Diabetes mellitus. Ergebn. allg. Path. path. Anat. 8, 538 (1902).

SCHLICHTKRULL, J.: Proinsulin und verwandte Proteine – chemische und biologische Untersuchungen. 76. Tagg Dtsch. Ges. Inn. Med., Wiesbaden 1970, p. 14. München: J. F. Bergmann 1970.

SCHMIDT, M. B.: Über die Beziehungen der Langerhansschen Inseln des Pankreas zum Diabetes mellitus. Münch. med. Wschr. 49, 51 (1902).

SEIFERT, G.: Die pathologische Morphologie der Langerhansschen Inseln, besonders beim Diabetes mellitus des Menschen. Verh. dtsch. Ges. Path. 42, 50 (1958).

SILVERMAN, J. O.: Eosinophile infiltration in the pancreas of infants of diabetic mothers. A clinicopathological study. Diabetes 12, 528 (1963).

SOLOMON, L. L., BLIZZARD, R. M.: Autoimmune disorders of endocrine glands. J. Pediat. 63 (1963).

SOMMERS, S. C.: Basement membranes, ground substance and lymphocytic aggregates in aging organs. J. Geront. 11, 251 (1956).

SPELLACY, W. N.: Human placental lactogen (HPL). The review of a protein hormone important to obstetrics and gynecology. Sth. med. J. (Bgham, Ala.) 62, 1054 (1969).

SPELLACY, W. N.: Plasma insulin, growth hormone and placental lactogen levels in normal and abnormal pregnancies. Acta endocr. (Kbh.), Suppl. 155, 82 (1971).

SSOBOLEFF, L. W.: Zur normalen und pathologischen Morphologie der inneren Sekretion der Bauchspeicheldrüse. Virchows Arch. Abt. A 168, 91 (1902).

STANSFIELD, O. H., WARREN, S.: Inflammation involving the islands of Langerhans in diabetes. New Engl. J. Med. 198, 686 (1928).

STANTON, E. R., JONES, H. W., MARBLE, A.: Coexisting diabetes mellitus and Addison's disease; observations and report of a case in a ten year-old boy. Arch. intern. Med. 93, 911 (1954).

STEINER, D. F., CHO, S., OYER, P. E., TERRIS, S., PETERSON, J. D., RUBENSTEIN, A. H.: Isolation and characterization of proinsulin C-peptide from bovine pancreas. J. biol. Chem. 246, 1365 (1970).

STEINER, D. F., HALLUND, O., RUBENSTEIN, A., CHO, S., BAYLISS, C.: Isolation and properties of proinsulin, intermediate forms and other minor components from crystalline bovine insulin. Diabetes 17, 725 (1968).

STEINER, D. F., OYER, P.: The biosynthesis of insulin and a probable precursor of insulin by a human islet cell adenoma. Proc. nat. Acad. Sci. (Wash.) 57, 473 (1967).

STEINER, H.: Insulitis beim perakuten Diabetes des Kindes. Klin. Wschr. 46, 417 (1968).

STEINKE, J., DRISCOLL, S. G.: The extractable insulin content of pancreas from fetuses and infants of diabetic and control mothers. Diabetes 14, 573 (1965).

TERBRÜGGEN, A.: Untersuchungen über Inselapparat -und Inseladenome, insbesondere über die Zelltypen bei Diabetes mellitus und Spontanhypoglykämie. Virchows Arch. Abt. A 315, 407 (1948).

THEMANN, H., ANDRA, J. A., ROSE, N. R., ANDRA, E. C., WITEBSKY, E.: Experimental thyroiditis in rhesus monkey. V. Electron microscopic investigations. Clin. exp. Immunol. 3, 491 (1968).

Toreson, W. E., Feldman, R., Lee, J. C., Grodsky, G. M.: Pathology of diabetes mellitus produced in rabbits by means of immunization with beef insulin. Amer. J. clin. Path. **42**, 531 (1964).

Toreson, W. E., Lee, J. C., Grodsky, G. M.: The histopathology of immune diabetes in the rabbit. Amer. J. Path. **52**, 1099 (1968).

Uhr, J. W., Salvin, S. B., Pappenheimer, A. M., Jr.: Induction of delayed hypersensitivity in guinea pigs by means of antigen-antibody complexes. J. exp. Med. **105**, 11 (1957).

Voisin, G. A.: Studies on experimental immunopathology of the spermatozoa and testicles. WHO, Scientific group on immunological aspects of human reproduction. Geneva, October 4–9 (1965).

Volk, B. W., Lazarus, S. S.: Ultramicroscopic evolution of B-cell ballooning degeneration in diabetic dogs. Lab. Invest. **12**, 697 (1963).

Volk, B. W., Lazarus, S. S., Wellmann, K. F.: Beta cell structure in latent and chronic diabetes of the rabbit. Diabetes **14**, 792 (1965).

Waksman, B. H.: A histologic study of the autoallergic testis lesion in the guinea pig. J. exp. Med. **109**, 311 (1959).

Waksman, B. H.: Animal investigations in autosensitization. Nervous system. Ann. N.Y. Acad. Sci. **124**, 299 (1965).

Waksman, B. H., Adams, R. D.: A comparative study of experimental allergic neuritis in the rabbit, guinea pig and mouse. J. Neuropath. exp. Neurol. **15**, 293 (1956).

Warren, S.: The pathology of diabetes in children. J. Amer. med. Ass. **88**, 99 (1927).

Warren, S., Le Compte, P. M.: The pathology of diabetes mellitus, p. 248–67. Philadelphia: Lea and Febiger 1952.

Warren, S., Le Compte, P. M., Legg, M. A.: The pathology of diabetes mellitus. Philadelphia: Lea and Febiger 1966.

Warren, S., Root, H. F.: The pathology of diabetes, with special reference to pancreatic regeneration. Amer. J. Path. **1**, 415 (1925).

Weichselbaum, A.: Über die Veränderungen des Pankreas beim Diabetes mellitus. S.-B. Akad. Wiss. Wien, math.-nat. Kl. **119**, 73 (1910).

Weichselbaum, A.: Über die Veränderungen des Pankreas beim Diabetes mellitus. Wien. klin. Wschr. **24**, 153 (1911).

Weigle, W. O.: The induction of autoimmunity in rabbits following injection of heterologous or altered homologous thyroglobulin. J. exp. Med. **121**, 289 (1965).

Witebsky, E., Rose, N. R., Terplan, K., Paine, J. R., Egan, R. W.: Chronic thyroiditis and autoimmunization. J. Amer. med. Ass. **164**, 1439 (1957).

Wright, P. H., Krisberg, R. A., Halpern, B., Dolkart, R. E.: Properties of insulin antibodies produced by the guinea pig, horse, sheep and man. Diabetes **11**, 519 (1962).

Yagi, Y., Maier, P., Pressman, D., Arbesman, C. E., Reisman, R. E., Lenzner, A. R.: Multiplicity of insulinbinding antibodies in human sera. J. Immunol. **90**, 760 (1963).

Institute of Pathology, University of Würzburg/Germany
(Director: Prof. Dr. H. W. Altmann)

Cytologic and Histologic Aspects of Toxically Induced Liver Reactions

O. KLINGE

With 8 Figures

Contents

I. Introduction

In recent years many attempts have been made to classify the commercially available substances and drugs which may have a toxic effect on the liver. The identified culprits have been compiled in lists (DÖLLE and MARTINI, 1959, 1962, 1964, 1966) and critically evaluated (POPPER and SCHAFFNER, 1959; SMETANA, 1963; KLATSKIN, 1963; POPPER et al., 1965; SHERLOCK, 1965, 1966, EDMONDSON and PETERS, 1967; LEVI, 1967; REMMER, 1969; STENGER, 1970). Their number seems to be still growing, however, and, in addition, numerous environmental substances may play a causative role. But even in the numerous cases where substances have been clearly identified as hepatotoxins and as responsible for the induction of badly defined clinical entities, morphological changes in the liver have received comparatively little attention. This might be partly due to the fact that in each individual case the specific injury is difficult to predict and to differentiate deliberately and is rarely defined. Actually, while a few substances, the so-called direct hepatotoxins, invariably lead to alterations of the liver parenchyma, most of the substances discussed here generally fail to do so, and direct incompatibility of drugs is rarely manifest. Etiological studies are therefore not only important, but decisive, since a causative therapy should not remain unspecific, as is often the case with inflammatory liver diseases. On the contrary, therapy must include the elucidation of the etiology of the disease, thus enabling the elimination of the responsible agent. Unfortunately, in most cases we are still far from this causal identification. Only a few substances or classes of substances can be associated with a defined pattern of hepatic alteration. Morphological studies, on the other hand, using purely cytological criteria, permit a certain rubrification of some of the resulting hepatic changes (KLINGE, 1969; KLINGE and ALTMANN, 1971; ALTMANN u. KLINGE, 1972). This cytological approach leads to the realization of two types of reactive patterns: one, a set of reactions which must be taken as indicative of an adaptive or compensatory process, caused by changes in the cellular metabolism; the second, a series of epithelial changes which in other lesions of the liver are rarely observed to the same degree or in the same combinations, and therefore serve as a fairly typical basic pattern of all known toxic alterations in the liver. Only against this background of cytological analysis can the changes on the next level, the histological one, be justly evaluated. Hepatocellular changes and histological reactions—celullar infiltration, activation of the mesenchyme and an increase in fiber formation—combine with each other to form a reasonable pattern. Only these combined patterns justify the distinction between drug-induced liver alterations as hepatoses and the various forms of hepatitis (KLINGE, 1969a), since primary inflammatory processes are usually not involved in hepatoses (SMETANA, 1963) and, if observed, are commonly due to secondary effects.

II. Cellular Adaptation Phenomena

Among adaptive processes, the increase in *agranular endoplasmic reticulum* within hepatocytes has attracted considerable attention in recent years. Under the light microscope a distinct cellular pattern can be observed, characterized by a fine granulation and an opacity of large areas within the cytoplasm as observed in hematoxylin-eosine preparations (Fig. 1 a). The nucleus is frequently functionally enlarged, that is, it shows a loose chromatin pattern, contains a large basophilic nucleolus, and is usually situated close to the cellular periphery. The basophilic ergastoplasmic granules seem to be forced into this zone (BRUNI, 1960). It has been well documented in experimental animals (PORTER and BRUNI, 1959; STEINER and BAGLIO, 1963; BANNASCH, 1968) that this light microscopic pattern corresponds to the electron microscopic observation of a dense network of tubular and vesicular structures of ribosome-free membranes. Occasionally these findings have been confirmed in human liver biopsies too (BIAVA and MUKHLOVA-MONTIEL, 1965; KLINGE and BANNASCH, 1968). Commonly a close topographical relationship exists between

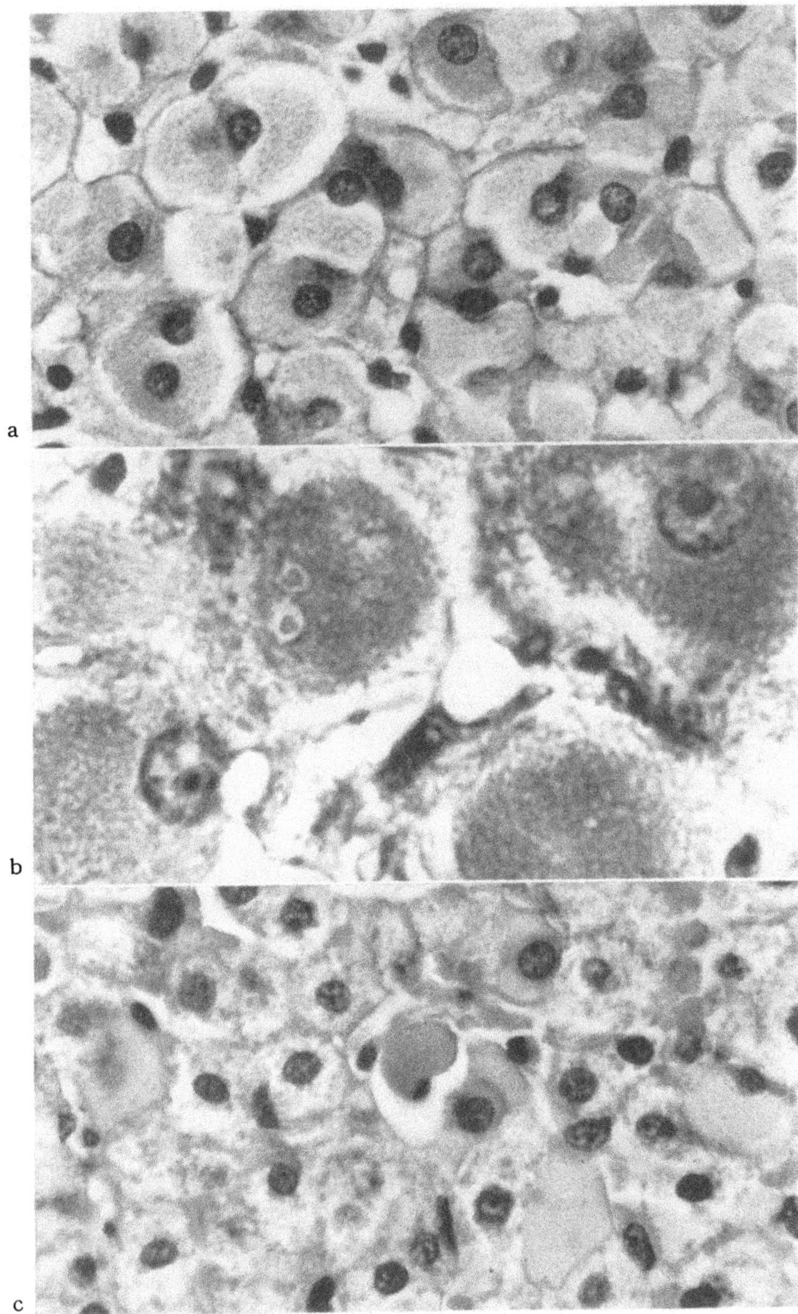

Fig. 1 a–c. Hypertrophic agranular endoplasmic reticulum following chronic alcoholism (a and b) and PAS medication for tuberculosis (c): Finest granular, opalescent foci of cytoplasm, pale eosinophilic in HE preparations (a and c) with apparently high glycogen content (b). Hyaline droplet inclusions within an agranular area (b). Transitions of cells with increased smooth membranes into coagulation necrosis (c). a and c hematoxylin-eosin, 990 × ; b Best's carmin, 1600 ×

increased smooth endoplasmic reticulum and finely granulated areas of glycogen storage (PORTER and BRUNI, 1959; BANNASCH and MÜLLER, 1964) (Fig. 1 b). This relationship is not necessarily a linear one, but usually the glycogen content is higher than that of normal liver cells. The reasons for these parallel changes in glycogen metabolism are so far poorly understood (STEINER and BAGLIO, 1963; ROUILLER, 1964; BANNASCH, 1968; STENGER, 1970). In normal liver cells smooth endoplasmic reticulum is visible only under the electron microscope, where drug-induced increase in lamellar structures also can be distinctly visualized within a short time after the onset of exposition (REMMER and MERKER, 1963; REMMER, 1965; SMUCKLER and ARCASOY, 1969). Under the light microscope, on the other hand, changes may only be observed after long-term administration of enzyme-inducing substances. The altered epithelia are diffusely distributed in the liver acini, arranged in small foci or accumulated in its central parts. Since proliferation of the system can, in principle, be evoked by all lipoid-soluble substances which are metabolized in liver cells (BURNS et al., 1963; REMMER, 1969; STENGER, 1970), this pattern is especially distinct in cases of chronic barbiturate abuse, after the administration of tuberculostatics, cytostatics, analgesics and oral antidiabetics (v. SEEBACH et al., 1972). A very pronounced increase in the smooth endoplasmic reticulum of almost all of the epithelia of a liver biopsy can occasionally be observed by the light microscope in cases of chronic alcoholism (KLINGE, 1971). Finally, hepatocytes whose cytoplasm is dominated by agranular endoplasmic reticulum are found in numerous cases of cirrhotic livers. This finding might be connected with an increased function of the remaining parenchyma; more likely it is due to the action of causal or accidental toxic injuries (KLINGE and BANNASCH, 1968). It seems important that the drug-induced proliferation of the smooth endoplasmic reticulum is reversible after cessation of drug administration (STENGER, 1970), while similar changes are irreversible when induced by a carcinogen (BANNASCH, 1968).

Another question concerns the actual significance of the increase in endoplasmic reticulum to a degree visible by light microscopy. Methods of conventional histology do not permit determination of whether the proliferation of the membrane structures reflects enhanced enzyme activity or whether the massive increase which leads to light optical visibility is due only to an increase in functionally inert cytoplasmic organelles. In other words, we may be observing hyperplastic but hypoactive membranous lamellae (SCHAFFNER and POPPER, 1969; HUTTERER et al., 1969). This view is supported by the fact that the rate of necrosis is usually higher in livers exhibiting a pronounced hypertrophy of the smooth endoplasmic reticulum, and that, occasionally, one observes transitions into coagulation necrosis in epithelia whose cytoplasm is dominated by agranular membranes (Fig. 1 c). In rare instances hyaline droplet inclusions can be demonstrated within the agranular areas (Fig. 1 b), probably indicating circumscribed zones of necrosis (ALBOT and JEZEQUEL, 1962; BIAVA and MUKHLOVA-MONTIEL, 1965), which might be equivalent to so-called "cytoplasmic whorls" seen in liver cells of experimental animals (ALTMANN and OSTERLAND, 1961). In addition, it is possible that a certain segment of the dense, eosinophilic protein droplets which are occasionally observed after the abuse of analgesics, especially Optalidon, and, even more frequently, in cases of chronic alcoholism, represent areas of coagulated smooth endoplasmic reticulum. They may correspond to the defined zones of necrosis observed in hepatoma cells whose origin from hyperplastic agranular endoplasmic reticulum can sometimes be demonstrated (KLINGE, 1971).

On the other hand, hyaline droplets in the cytoplasm are morphogenetically not uniform. This nonuniformity is evidenced by the fact that under the electron microscope they sometimes look like giant mitochondria (e.g. WILSON and LEDUC, 1963; SVOBODA and HIGGINSON, 1963; ERICSSON *et al.*, 1966; RUBIN and LIEBER, 1968), especially in chronic alcoholism (SVOBODA and MANNING, 1964; ISERI and GOTTLIEB, 1971). Protein droplets which are indistinguishable by light microscopy from the above mentioned ones may also be associated with lysosomal processes and occur in cases of the so-called *lipofuscinosis* (LUND and OLSEN, 1970) of the liver. Here, exceptionally coarsely granulated deposits of lipopigments can be observed and, occasionally, pure protein droplets (Fig. 2a) which are caused by long-term abuse of phenacetine-, pyramidone-, and acetylsalicyl acid containing analgesics (ABRAHAMS *et al.*, 1964; STUDER and SCHÄRER, 1965; BERNEIS and STUDER, 1967, 1968; HAUDENSCHILD, 1969). The histological evidence is striking, both concerning the topography of the pigmented epithelia and the content of pigment in an individual cell (Fig. 3a). The substance can be demonstrated in liver epithelia at the center of the lobule, in intermediary and, sometimes, even in acinus-peripheral positions. The individual cell may often be overloaded with small or coarse inhomogenous particles (Fig. 3) and also with round droplet-shaped protein deposits (Fig. 2a). The coarsely granulated depository forms are particularly indicative. The shape of the granules and their abundance may evoke patterns similar to those observed histomorphologically in the liver in the Dubin-Johnson syndrome (SAMIOS *et al.*, 1965; BARONE *et al.*, 1969) and clearly distinguish the phenomenon from the usual form of lipofuscin observed in elderly patients (PORTA and HARTROFT, 1969). Except for this difference, methods available today do not permit one to differentiate between pigment induced by phenacetin and that resulting from age. Background-fluorescence in unstained preparations (Fig. 3b), argentaffinity (Fig. 3c) and positive reactions for proteins, lipids and fatty acids (Fig. 3d), all point to the lipofuscin character of the inhomogenous substance. Occasionally, a lipoid nucleus is surrounded by a protein coat (BERNEIS and STUDER, 1967, 1968; HAUDENSCHILD and STUDER, 1971), which corresponds to the pattern observed under the electron microscope, where, in addition to proteins, lipoids and neutral fats, coarse residual bodies equivalent to the granules dominate the picture (ABRAHAMS *et al.*, 1964).

The cytoplasm of cells which are loaded with pigment is sometimes also characterized by an increase in smooth endoplasmic reticulum which is poorly

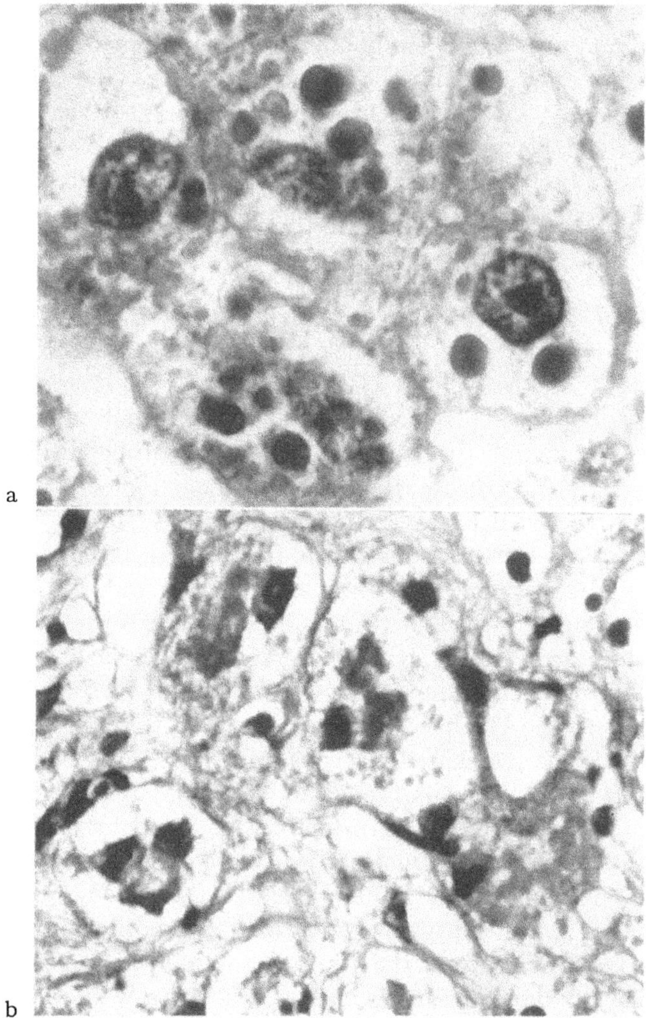

Fig. 2 a and b. Hyaline cytoplasma inclusions, a Large protein droplets of variable density caused by chronic phenacetine medication in an asthmatic. b Bizarrely shaped inhomogeneous deposits of so-called alcoholic hyaline and its precursors (bottom right). a Goldner's trichrome staining, 1600 × ; b hematoxylin-eosin, 990 ×

discernible under the light microscope, but quite pronounced under the electron microscope (PFEIFER, personal communication). This increase of the drug-metabolizing system may be partially responsible for the occurrence of the myelin-figures seen in electron microscopic pictures of the granules. The less striking effect observed under the light microscope versus the more pronounced one seen under the electron microscope might indicate an enhanced turnover of smooth membranes in the presence of high concentrations of the substrate (HAUDEN-SCHILD, 1969). This, however, does not satisfactorily explain cell pigmentation. Additional factors, e.g. an inhibition of lysosomal autophagy

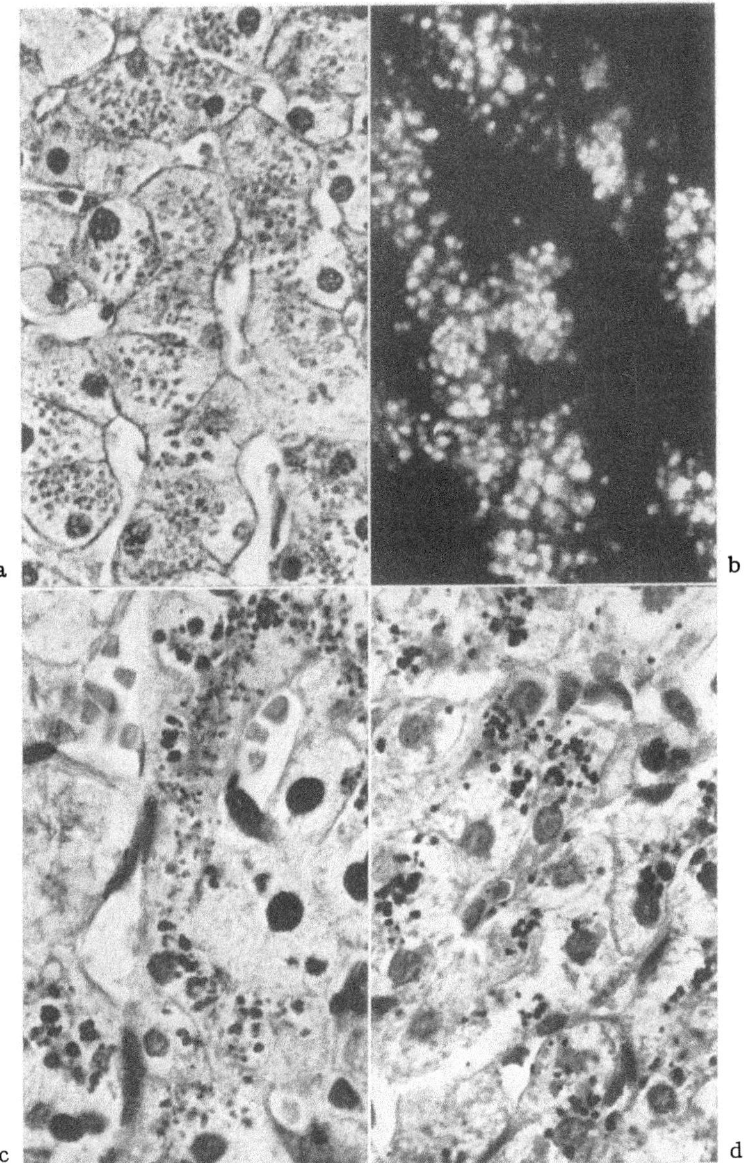

Fig. 3a–d. Lipofuscinosis after long-lasting Pyramidone abusus: Abundant inhomogeneous coarse granules within the cytoplasm of intermediary liver epithelium (a), showing fluorescence in unstained preparations (b), positive argentaffinity (c), and reactions for fatty acids (d). a hematoxylin-eosin, 660 × ; b fluorescence-preparation, 660 × ; c Masson-Hamperl, 990 × ; d Ziehl-Neelsen, 990 ×

(TORHORST *et al.*, 1967), must play a decisive role in the massive accumulation of degradation products. A slightly increased rate of necrosis indicates parenchymal changes (KLINGE and ALTMANN, 1971). Finally, individual factors may be important, since not all patients with phenacetine-induced interstitial nephritis show pigmentation of the hepatocytes. In other cases the accumulation of granules in the liver cell is predominant without clinical manifestation of lesions in the kidney. One may conclude that, as in the case of other toxic injuries, genetic factors may influence the reactions induced by phenacetine abuse or be responsible for their organ manifestation.

III. Alterative Epithelial Lesions

Changes which become manifest primarily as lesions of the hepatic parenchyma fall into certain basic patterns. They usually occur concomitantly, but in rare cases may be seen in pure form. As such they shall be briefly outlined.

1. Intrahepatic Cholestasis

Cholestasis of noninflammatory hepatic origin, when present in its massive form, may histomorphologically give rise to significant difficulties in differential diagnosis. In biopsies there is actually no reliable criterion which would permit one to differentiate in all cases toxic cholestasis from incomplete obstructive icterus. Electron microscopy is of no great help either (SCHAFFNER and SASAKI, 1965). In most cases, however, discrimination is possible on the basis of several impressive changes: biliary deposits are predominantly found in the center of the lobule, as intraepithelial droplets or, more frequently and in many cases even more pronounced (KLINGE, 1971), as intercellular thrombi. The cytoplasm of liver epithelia afflicted by cholestasis is, as a rule, characteristically altered. With variable frequency, it may be more or less light (see DOONER et al., 1971); the basophilic ergastoplasm is concentrated in the vicinity of the interepithelial canaliculi (Fig. 4a), which can be clearly observed after elective staining of nucleic acids (Fig. 4b). The displacement of the basophilic ergastoplasm may be taken as indicative of an active accumulation of the organelles in the vicinity of canaliculi (ALTMANN, 1955; KLINGE, 1965). This would be a morphological indication that in drug-induced cholestasis both lesions of the cell membrane and their excretional function dominate over possible disturbances of intracellular uncoupling processes. Even detailed scrutiny does not provide any evidence for the latter. In contrast to extrahepatic cholestasis, intrahepatic cholestasis does not lead to dilatation of the preformed biliary ducts. In uncomplicated cases which are biopsied early, the cholangioles are intact and not proliferated, which may facilitate differential diagnosis. Almost as a rule, diffusely distributed necrosis of a variable number of single cells is observed.

Intrahepatic cholestasis has long been known as icterus in pregnancy (HAEMMERLI, 1966) and therefore its increasing frequency as a side-effect of the use of ovulation inhibitors for birth control is not surprising (e.g. POPPER and SCHAFFNER, 1959; CULLBERG et al., 1965; LARSSON-COHN and STENRAM, 1965; v. OLDERSHAUSEN et al., 1965; POPPER et al., 1965; THULIN and NERMARK 1966; SHERLOCK, 1966). In both instances, i.e. pregnancy and the contra-

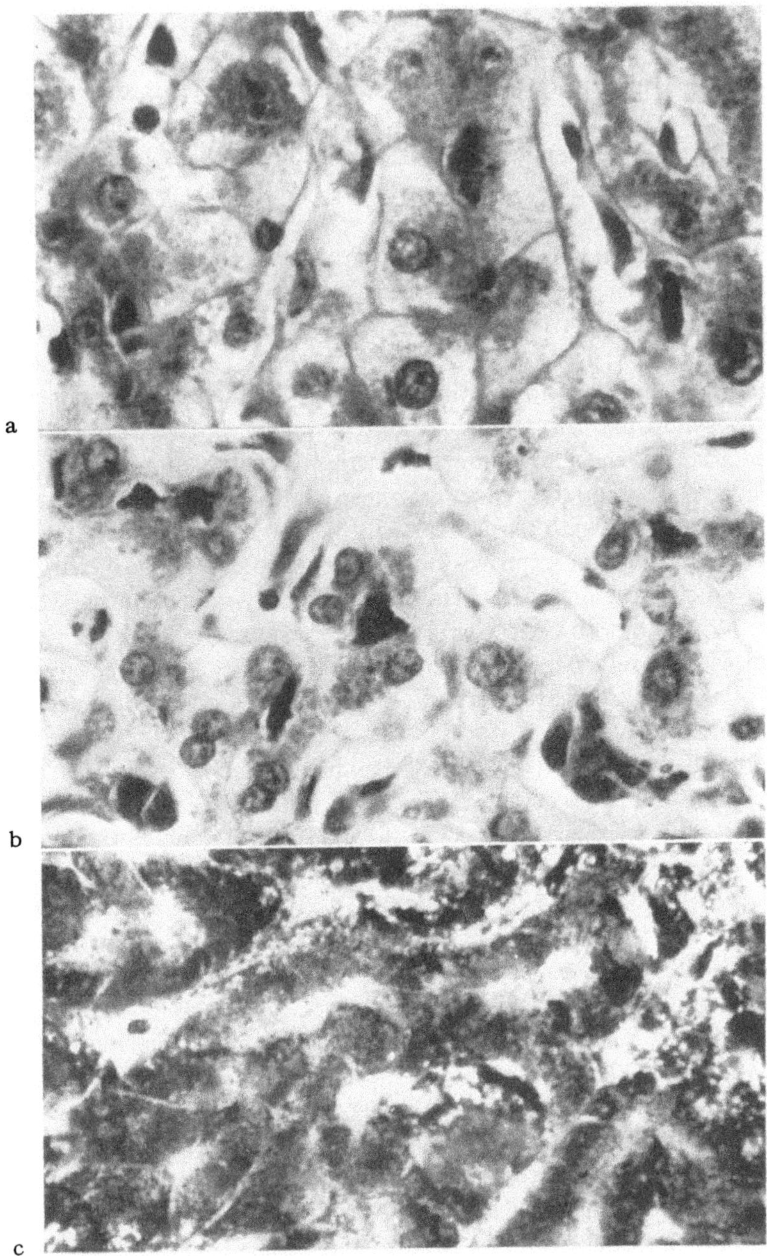

a

b

c

Fig. 4a–c. Intrahepatic cholestasis as a side-effect of contraceptives: Intraepithelial bile droplets and — more often — intercellular bile thrombi. Concentration of the baso-philic ergastoplasm in the vicinity of the canaliculi leading to light peripherial cytoplasm appearance (a and b) parallel with epithelial glycogen storage in the light regions (c). a hematoxylin-eosin, b Kresylviolett, c Tri-PAS-reaction, 990 ×

ceptive pill, intrahepatic cholestasis is induced by high concentrations (SHERLOCK, 1965; LEVI, 1967) of steroids which carry an α-keto-group at the C-17 position, that is, the estrogens (DRILL, 1963; ARIAS, 1963; KRÜSKEMPER and NOELL, 1967; CACHIN, 1967). Drug-induced cholestasis offers the analysis of two interesting points: First, women suffering from toxic cholestasis when taking ovulation inhibitors also usually suffer from icterus during gravidity (HAEMMERLI and WYSS, 1967). This points towards—or almost proves—some individual enzyme deficiency. A genetic component is also suggested by the fact that the jaundice observed after the use of ovulation inhibitors showed high regional frequencies both in Scandinavia (e.g. CULLBERG et al., 1965) and in Chile (ORELLANA-ALCALDE and DOMINGUEZ, 1966). On the other hand, rare cases have been observed with improvement of the icterus in spite of uninterrupted administration of the responsible drug, phenothiacine in these instances (AYD, 1963; EDMONDSON and PETERS, 1967; LEVI, 1967). Also, not all patients who succumb to the disease after primary exposure relapse when exposed a second time (SHERLOCK, 1966). Obviously, in these cases the above-mentioned adaptive mechanism in the glucoronylating system of the agranular endoplasmic reticulum becomes manifest, but does so with retardation (KLINGE and ALTMANN, 1971). No rule can be given, however, and in general, the drug-induced icterus improves only after discontinuation of the inducing agent, in some cases, however, persisting for weeks and months (HURT and WEGMAN, 1961; NØRREDAM, 1963). Such severe symptoms of toxic cholestatic liver injuries not only occur in steroid treatment (SCHAFFNER et al., 1959; GILBERT et al., 1963) but are especially typical of the phenothiazines (POPPER and SCHAFFNER, 1959; AYD, 1963; KLATSKIN, 1963; SMETANA, 1963; SHERLOCK, 1964, 1966; POPPER et al., 1965) and this whole group of drugs. Even though chlorpromazine induces very severe cases of cholestasis which may persist for months or even years (NØRREDAM, 1963; COOK and SHERLOCK, 1965, 1966), the truth again holds that individual tolerance varies tremendously (POPPER and SCHAFFNER, 1959; SMETANA, 1963; POPPER et al., 1965; LEVI, 1967). Above all, the injury usually is not permanent and critical evaluation of the literature (MEYERS et al., 1957; POPPER, 1958; HURT and WEGMANN, 1961; KOHN and MYERSON, 1961; WALKER and COMBES, 1966) makes it doubtful that primary biliary cirrhosis is induced by phenothiazine (SHERLOCK, 1965; KLINGE and ALTMANN, 1971). The doubt is the more justified since drug-induced cholestasis usually follows a rather benign course (v. OLDERSHAUSEN, 1968), regardless of which of the possible inducers causes it: steroids lacking the α-keto-group at C-17, cytostatics, antidiabetics, antibiotics, antidepressives, antipsychotics or antiepileptics (KLINGE and ALTMANN, 1971b). The same holds true for those cases of intrahepatic cholestasis which appear as the first warning signal in adolescent alcoholics, without as yet showing any further parenchymal changes under the light microscope (KLINGE, 1971).

2. Toxic Cell Swelling

The pattern of toxic cell swelling (KLINGE, 1969a)—often discrete and perhaps for this reason rarely taken into consideration—shows morphological features similar to intrahepatic cholestasis. It manifests itself in a displacement

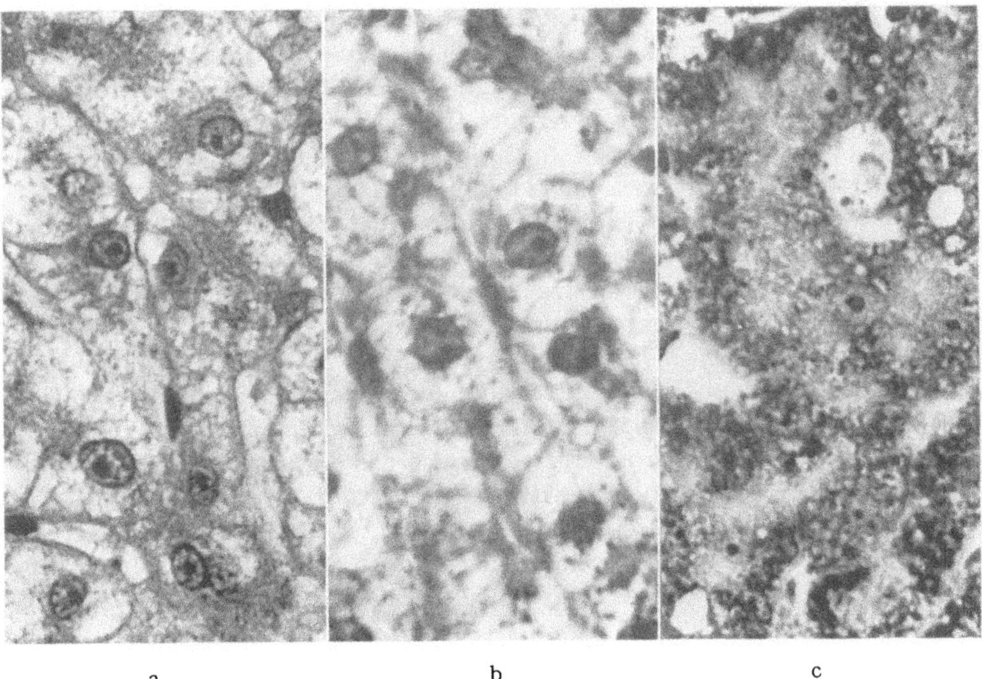

a   b   c

Fig. 5 a–c. Toxic cell swelling in the course of continued PAS medication (a), Trichlor-etylene intoxication (b) and chronic alcoholism (c). Discrete concentration of the baso-philic ergastoplasm towards the biliary epithelial pole (a and b) combined with striking accumulation of glycogen within the sinusoidal cell region. a hematoxylin-eosin, b Kre-sylviolett, c Best's carmin, 990 ×

of ribosome studded basophilic endoplasmic reticulum towards the peribiliar cell pole (Fig. 5 a). In contrast to intrahepatic cholestasis, this regional con-centration of the cytoplasmic organelles seems to be associated with their degradation. This is evidenced by the fact that staining of the cell with baso-philic dyes is reduced everywhere, not just at the periphery of the cell (KLINGE and ALTMANN, 1971 b) (Fig. 5 b). The striking clearing of the cytoplasm in the vicinity of the sinusoidal cell pole is the second characteristic of this kind of injury (Fig. 5 a+b). One at first is led to the assumption that one is dealing with hydropic swelling of the epithelia (SMETANA, 1963; EDMONDSON and PETERS, 1967). However, in most cases one can show histochemically that the above observation is based on the intraepithelial accumulation of poly-saccharides. They may in most cases even be demonstrated if the biopsy material has been fixed in formalin (Fig. 5 c), although this kind of fixation leads to partial loss of glycogen from the tissue. The congruence between the so-called hydropic swelling of the cell and the intense intracytoplasmatic glycogen storage is well documented in the case of experimental carcinogenesis (BANNASCH and MÜLLER, 1964; BANNASCH, 1968). There, however, polysac-charide storage occurs diffusely over the entire cell, not only at the sinusoidal pole. Also, the effect is irreversible in experimental carcinogenesis, while in the known cases of intoxication of the human liver, glycogen storage seems to be reversible once administration of the inducing substance is discontinued. The changes are highly characteristic; they may be due to an interference with the utilization of glycogen which would still be synthesized but no longer secreted or, if so, only to a limited extent (KLINGE and ALTMANN, 1971 a). This effect could either be brought about by a deranged enzyme system or by changes in membrane transport. Even though the pathogenesis is doubtful, this kind of glycogen storage together with the displacement of basophilic ergastoplasm may serve as a sure criterion for toxin-induced metabolic changes, next to fatty infiltration of the epithelium. It is the joint appearance of cellular displacement of basophilic material and glycogen storage which leads to the characteristic epithelial aspect observed in intrahepatic cholestasis (Fig. 4c). Because the phenomenon is often accompanied by a marked enlargement of the cell, one may generally designate this form as a toxic cell swelling. Changes occur primarily in areas located towards the center of the acini, though occasionally, they are confined to small sectors or are diffusely distributed. They are induced by a wide variety of toxic substances and are thus—together with fat storage of the parenchyma—the most frequently encountered alteration. Among occupational hazards, halogenated hydrocarbon derivatives are especially potent in inducing this pattern. It is also frequently seen in chronic alcoholism and with equal frequency in cases of drug-incompatibility. We observed this pattern after therapy with tuberculostatics, glycerole-derivatives, anabolic steroids, anticonvulsives, sedatives, analgesics (see SMETANA, 1963; EDMONDSON and PETERS, 1967) and halothane anesthesia (see PETERS et al., 1969). It is likely, however, that this list is far from complete.

3. Fatty Infiltration of Epithelia

Our knowledge of the etiology of toxic fatty liver degeneration is still quite uncertain. Usually alcohol is blamed. Cortisone and its derivatives (SCHMID-BIRCHER, 1954; DONTENWILL et al., 1955; BÄSSLER, 1961; GILBERT et al., 1963) and, occasionally, phenylbutazone (ECKER, 1965) and tetracycline seem to be the main culprits among medicaments. Two types of fatty infiltration of the parenchyma can be observed: the more frequent one manifests itself in the form of middle or coarsely shaped droplets; the altered epithelia are either diffusely distributed over the lobules or grouped into defined zones. Our experience shows that in particular the mixture of different sizes of droplets indicates a toxic etiology (Fig.6a). Similar findings are obtained after amanita poisoning, after treatment with tuberculostatics, cytostatics, antibiotics (ROBINSON and SEAKINS, 1962), or, after a single lethal dose of halothane-anesthesia and in transitory halothane injuries (KLINGE 1965, lit., 1972). The second type of fatty infiltration is characterized by uniformly diffuse fat deposits in microdroplets, leading to a foamy appearance of

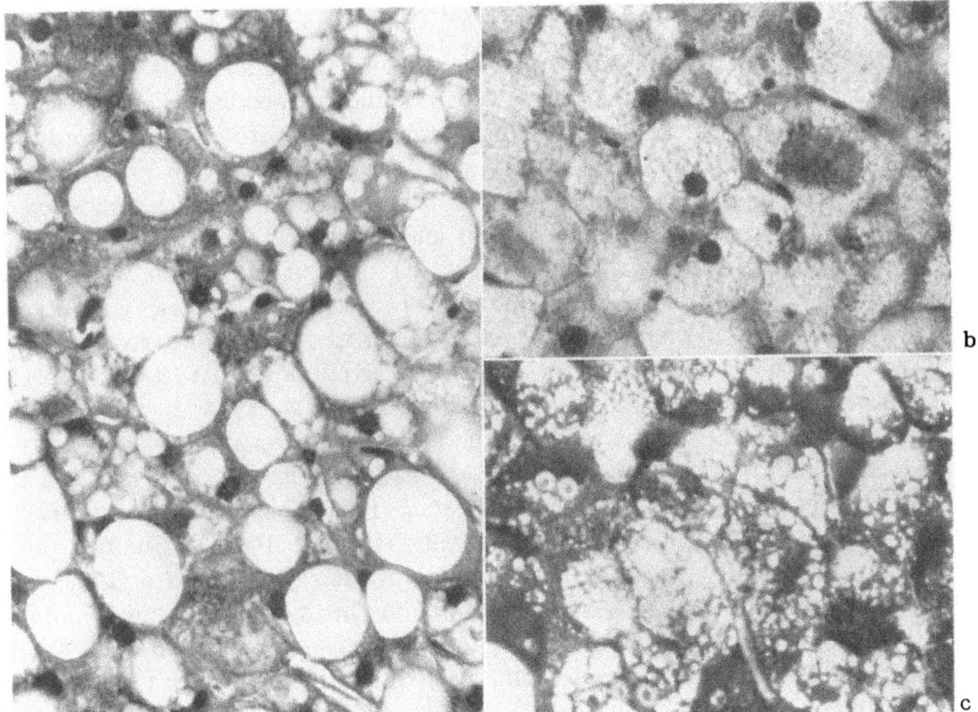

Fig. 6a–c. Fatty infiltration: Mixture of droplets of variable sizes after halothane anaesthesia (a). Ultrafine-foamy form in an acute alcoholic intoxication (b and c) with coincidental signs of toxic cell swelling by glycogen accumulation. a and b hematoxylin-eosin, c Tri-PAS-reaction, 375 ×

the cytoplasm (Fig. 6b). It is a special characteristic of a highly acute or acutely intensified intoxication, which explains why this form is occasionally encountered in chronic alcoholism (see STENGER, 1970). For endogenous and for the most part unknown reasons, the most severe, often lethal cases of acute fatty liver metamorphosis of the above-described type occur in pregnancy (SHEEHAN, 1940; PETERS et al., 1962; HARMS, 1966; KÜHN et al., 1967). This type has also been described after treatment with tetracycline (SCHULTZ et al., 1963; PETERS et al., 1967; STENGER, 1970), especially during pregnancy (KUNELIS et al., 1965; EDMONDSON and PETERS, 1967). Both forms of toxic fatty infiltration, whether characterized by the ultrafine or the mixed droplet type, are frequently accompanied by peribilial concentration of basophilic ergastoplasm (Fig. 6c). Thus, they show some of the characteristics of toxic cell swelling, especially since glycogen storage at the capillaries may also be encountered. Still, the pathogenesis of fatty infiltration of the epithelia is often obscure, possibly taking different routes. It is likely that it depends on the specific action of the individual drug or its metabolic products on the cellular lipoid- and protein metabolism (STENGER, 1970).

4. Parenchymal Necrosis

Cell death in the liver is observed morphologically in all kinds of injuries, either as coagulation necrosis, the so-called Councilman bodies (Fig. 7b), or as cytolyses or their precursor stages: pale, swollen cells with indistinct borders and prekaryolytic nuclei. Such forms per se are insufficient to prove toxic etiology; in general one must search for additional evidence of intoxication. Significant insight may be gained from leukocytic degradation processes of either individual cells or cell groups (Fig. 7c), even if they occur within an otherwise unaltered parenchyma. This type of scattered cell necrosis is induced by a variety of drugs (Popper and Schaffner, 1959; Smetana, 1963; Klatskin, 1963; Sherlock, 1964, 1965, 1966; Klinge and Altmann, 1971). The list runs from several antipyretics (Engleman et al., 1954; Mauer, 1955; Becker, 1965) some sulfonamides (Lederer and Rosenblatt, 1942; Herbut and Scaricaciottoli, 1945; More et al., 1946), antibiotics (Lepper et al., 1951; Lowell, 1955; Valdivia-Barriga et al., 1963), tuberculostatics (Cohen and Lawrence, 1957; Sleeper et al., 1960; Heymer, 1962; Moulding and Goldstein, 1962; Kuntz et al., 1967) and cytostatics (Doljanski and Rosin, 1944; Clarke et al., 1953) Gerhartz, 1961) to the monoaminooxidase inhibitors (Popper, 1958; Shay and Sun, 1958; Spellberg and Frankel, 1962), anticonvulsives (Schnabel and Lahl, 1964; Edmondson and Peters, 1967) and narcotics (Affolter et al., 1964; Klinge, 1965; Nissen, 1965).

It is still a question whether Mallory's bodies, which are highly characteristic of exogenous and endogenous intoxications, are part of this pattern. That is, are these bodies indeed focal zones of cytoplasmic degradation as might be suggested by their light microscopic appearance as inhomogenous, bizarrely shaped eosinophilic areas (Fig. 2b)? Alternatively, they may represent the condensation of denatured proteins (Iseri and Gottlieb, 1971). Under the electron microscope, the substance seems to consist of fibrous material of variable density apparently not surrounded by membranes (Biava, 1964; Flax and Tisdale, 1964; Smuckler, 1968; Iseri and Gottlieb, 1971). Correspondingly, under the light microscope alcoholic hyaline contrasts with the surroundings to various degrees. Greater aggregates seem to be the consequence of confluence of small particles. The presence of Mallory's bodies is usually considered a bad prognostic sign in severe cases of chronic alcoholism. However, both light- and electron microscopy may reveal similar structures in further exogenous and endogenous, toxically-induced hepatoses. So-called alcoholic hyaline may, for instance, be observed in cases of primary biliar cirrhosis, in infantile cirrhosis (Nayak et al., 1969; Smetana et al., 1971) and, in our own experience, in peliosis hepatis. In all of these cases, the existent icterus may well be the tertium comparationis. Such intracytoplasmic inclusions have also been observed in morbus Wilson (Popper, 1968) and in hepatomas (Ishak and Grunz, 1967; Norkin and Campagna-Pinto, 1968).

Zonal parenchymal defects, in their pure form, either indicate a previous severe circulatory collapse or provide almost definite proof for the tran-

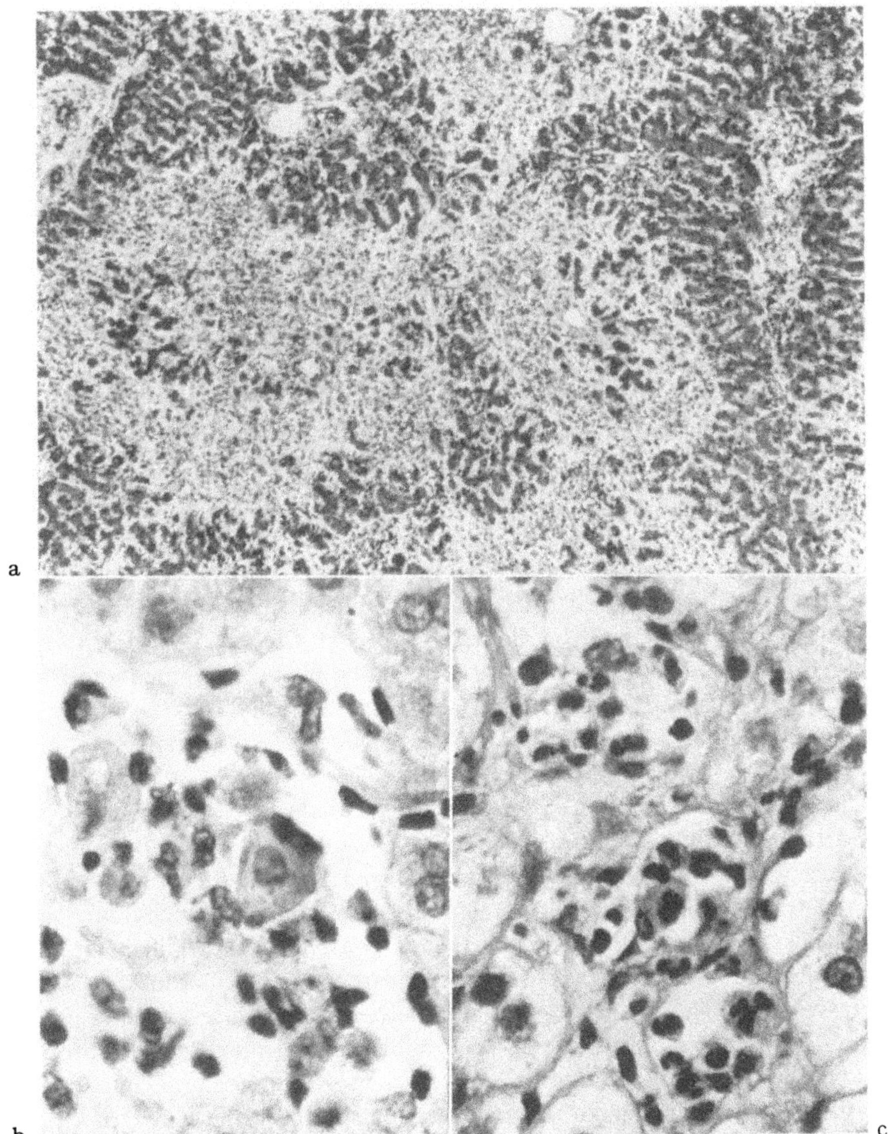

Fig. 7a–c. Parenchymal necrosis. Acute subtotal necrosis of liver epithelia after halothane anaesthesia leaving only a small peripherial margin of cells alive (a). Councilman bodies with surrounding Kupffer cell reaction following cytostatic therapy (b). Leukocytic degradation processes in the course of anticonvulsive medication. a–c hematoxylin-eosin. a 120 ×, b and c 990 ×

sitory action of a potent toxin. In early biopsied cases one observes an empty, loosely structured reticulin framework. The meshwork may include increased numbers of erythrocytes. Later, Kupffer's cells accumulate along the borders of the damaged areas (Fig. 7b). The cytoplasm of these cells is swollen and loaded with phagocytosed degraded pigment which originates from decaying liver cells (ALTMANN, 1970). In some cases clumps of Kupffer's cells take the place of the lost parenchyma. In their classic forms, such necrotic foci occur in amanita poisoning at the center of the lobule, in acidic acid poisoning at the periphery. Similar effects have been observed in cases of industrial poisoning (SMETANA, 1963), for instance with carbon tetrachloride (KLATSKIN, 1963; HOSCHEK, 1969), phosphorus (SALFELDER *et al.*, 1966) and with various solvents used for synthetic polymers (e.g. dimethylformamide: MASSMANN, 1956; REINL and URBAN, 1965; see HOFMAN, 1961). In addition, focal necrosis may be found in cases of drug incompatibility, e.g. after the administration of cytostatics (MEACHAM *et al.*, 1952; URAM *et al.*, 1956), sulfonamides (BLOODWORTH, 1963), antipyretics (NATHAN *et al.*, 1953; FRASER, 1955; FISHER, 1960), narcotics (AFFOLTER *et al.*, 1964; KLINGE, 1965; PETERS *et al.*, 1969) and, in our own experience, after the use of psychosedatives. Such focal necrosis is basically an abortive form of an acute liver dystrophy which indeed has been described as a consequence of intoxication with phalloidin and carbon tetrachloride, but which may also be found after halothane-anesthesia (Fig. 7a) and the administration of phenylhydatoine-containing drugs. POPPER (POPPER *et al.*, 1965) has given a further list of responsible substances. Morphologically, this acute dystrophy cannot be distinguished from the one following an infection with the hepatitis virus, which has led such forms to be characterized as "hepatitis-like" (see POPPER *et al.*, 1965; SHERLOCK, 1966). One must, however, keep in mind that inflammatory processes do not participate in the essence of the histologic pattern.

The discussion of focal necrosis already exceeds the scope of the cytological alterations discussed here initially. The same would hold true for those rare cases where damage of the liver parenchyma is followed by a loss of their reticulin framework. Thus peliosis hepatis occurs in its parenchymal variant (GORDON *et al.*, 1960), the damaged zones being empty or filled with large masses of blood, sometimes exceeding the entire area of a liver lobule (YANOFF and RAWSON, 1964). One may question whether drugs are by themselves sufficient to lead to these alterations, or if a high intrasinusoidal pressure is an unavoidable pathogenetic factor, as previously discussed. The occasional involvement of medicaments is, however, suggested by the fact that cases of peliosis have been observed after administration of norethandrolone (KLITZEN and SILNY, 1960; GORDON *et al.*, 1960; YANOFF and RAWSON, 1964). Here, additional doses of cortisone (BHAGWAT and DEODHAR, 1968) may be an important contributing factor because of their negative influence on the maintenance and new formation of the reticulin framework (KLINGE and ALTMANN, 1971).

Another rarity is intrahepatic venal thrombosis and, consequently Budd-Chiari syndrome, following parenchymal necrosis, expecially under the influence of senecio alkaloids (BRAS and McLEAN, 1963). Identical aspects have further been reported after the use of cytostatics (HILL and JÜNGST, 1969) or of ovulation inhibitors (see ROTHWELL-JACKSON, 1968; GRAYSON and REILLY, 1968; CLUBB and GILES, 1968; ASBECK *et al.*, 1972). That hormonal treatment may present an important pathogenetic factor is further supported by the increased incidence of the Budd-Chiari syndrome during gravidity (BRUNTSCH *et al.*, 1958); and after oral contraceptives (BECKER and MOSER, 1967; CLUBB and GILES, 1968; but: KRASS, 1968).

5. Nuclear Alterations

In contrast to the typical alterations occurring in the cytoplasm as a consequence of toxic injury, nuclear changes are commonly uncharacteristic. The number of double nucleic cells frequently exceeds that which is characteristic of the specific age group (ALTMANN *et al.*, 1966). Furthermore, the percentage of large polyploid nuclei and of intranuclear cytoplasmic inclusions can increase. This is due to the fact that necrosis acts as a regenerative stimulus which, however, cannot manifest itself properly under the influence of the toxin. Mitotic alterations and disturbances are the result, leading to an altered distribution and shape of the nuclei (ALTMANN, 1966; KLINGE, 1969b). However, such effects are due to a variety of injuries and not only to toxic ones.

Chronic lead poisoning, on the other hand, may induce a fairly typical karyological phenomenon: inside the karyoplasm eosinophilic nuclear inclusions of various sizes are found. In contrast to the common cytoplasmic inclusions, they are not surrounded by membranes (KLINGE, 1970) in the karyoplasm. Besides lead poisoning, they may be induced in experimental animals by long-term application of bismuth. In humans, they are known in certain viral infections (MÜLLER, 1966).

The spectrum of isolated pathologic cellular alterations is now reviewed. It is relatively small but still lends some color to the histopathological patterns in toxic hepatoses, since a variety of combinations may be found. In other words, fatty infiltration, cell swelling, cholestasis and necrosis can be combined to various degrees. Hyaline droplets, alcoholic hyalin, an increase in smooth endoplasmic reticulum and altered karyotypes add variation and accent to the general patterns. The mentioned hepatocellular adaptation and alteration phenomena are of variable importance for differential diagnosis: Thus, lipofuscinosis and the increase in smooth endoplasmic reticulum are highly significant, toxic cell swelling and intrahepatic cholestasis are important, while most forms of fatty infiltration are of low diagnostic value. Finally, necrosis and especially single cell necrosis, by themselves, rarely permit one to decide whether they are caused by a primary toxic injury or by some other mechanism.

IV. Histological Reactions

During the acute stage of toxic liver injuries, histological reactions are comparatively small (SMETANA, 1963). They are usually confined to defined removing processes, partially caused by leukocytes, partially by locally proliferating Kuppfer cells. There is no diffuse activation of the mesenchyme nor is there a significant cellular infiltration in the portal triads. These facts indicate that primary inflammation is not involved and that inflammatory reactions are not a prerequisite for toxic hepatosis. It therefore seems useful to summarize toxin-induced liver cell injuries under the term "toxic hepatoses", thus separating them from primary inflammatory lesions, i.e., from the various forms of hepatitis (KLINGE, 1969a).

Reactions on the histologic level may, of course, to various degrees add to and modify the ensuing picture. Additional changes may for instance be observed relatively early in the course of drug-induced cholestasis (SHERLOCK, 1964) at the portal areas. Here severe edema is manifest and by the loosening and aqueous impregnation of the portal tissue, the biliary ducts become distinctly pronounced. Concomitantly, one observes cellular infiltration, especially with eosinophilic leukocytes (SHERMAN, 1949; POPPER and SCHAFFNER, 1959; SHERLOCK, 1964; EDMONDSON and PETERS, 1967). This pattern has therefore been termed "eosinophilic cholangitis". The name might imply an allergic component in or even the allergic etiology of these alterations, both at the portal field and in the parenchyma (POPPER and SCHAFFNER, 1959; SLEEPER et al., 1960; STEINER, 1961; VALDIVIA-BARRIGA et al., 1963; ECKER, 1965). However, similar eosinophilic infiltrations in the triads may be observed in cases where there is certainly no allergic involvement, as in extrahepatic cholestasis, and even in cases of alcoholism. Inflammatory lesions of intrahepatic biliary ducts are certainly neither the primary reason nor a contributing factor in the latter cases of cholestasis; on the other hand severe eosinophilic reactions in blood, parenchyma and triads may be indicative of an allergic condition, as especially observed in halothane-induced lesions (PETERS et al., 1969; KLINGE, 1972). Within the parenchyma one observes enhanced mesenchymal reactions around individual necrotic cells; the reactions, however, remain quite localized. In some cases of chronic intoxication, a moderately diffuse activity of Kupper's cells has been reported; it is often accompanied by the appearance of phagocytosed erythrocytes and an ensuing siderosis in such cells; the pattern has been described in some cases of industrial intoxications and, mainly, in chronic alcoholism; it is especially pronounced in complicated cases, e.g. during the manifestation of a Zieve syndrome and its abortive forms (KLINGE, 1969a, 1971). Where widespread lesions of parenchyma precede, one actually observes the formation of intralobular granulomas which sometimes contain epithelioid cells or even eosinophilic leukocytes; this has been observed after intoxication with sulfonamides (MOORE et al., 1946; TISDALE, 1958), sulfanyl-urea (BLOODWORTH, 1963) and phenylbutazone (GOLDSTEIN, 1963). Even in such cases, though, the primary toxic character of the lesions remains easily identifiable.

Clarity and certainty of the diagnosis, however, may become endangered in the later course of toxic hepatosis. In severe cases, in which considerable amounts of cell debris and cell fragments are drained rather early into the lymphoid vessels of the portal fields, one frequently observes an increased cellular infiltration within the fields which may sometimes extend towards the parenchyma (Fig. 8). When this happens, a definite diagnosis may become

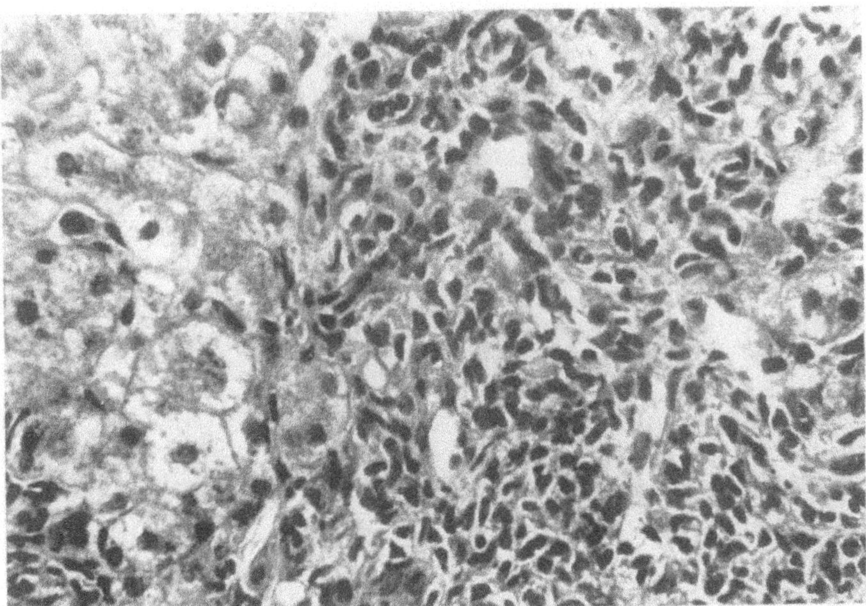

Fig. 8. Cellular infiltration and fiber formation of a portal triad in the course of tuber-culostatic therapy lasting two years, similar to the alterations in chronic hepatitis. Discrete toxic cell swelling of the adjacent epithelia is still visible. hematoxylin-eosin, 480 ×

difficult. As chronic intoxications progress further, the observations made in the parenchyma become less and less characteristic and, accordingly, altera-tions in the periphery become predominant. Finally, the resulting patterns become barely or completely indiscernible from those observed in chronic hepatitis (Fig. 8), especially since the process is increasingly accompanied by additional fiber formation within the portal fields and in their vicinity (URAM et al., 1956; NIEDOBITEK, 1968; HILL and JÜNGST, 1969; KOHN and MONTES, 1969). One further observes a condensation of the reticulin fibers, either because the lymph flow within the spaces of Disse, leading to the portal lymphoid vessels, is rendered more difficult or because activation or functional alteration of the Kupffer cells is accompanied by increased deposition of muco-polysaccharides at the reticulin framework. The last process, in any case, seems to be of some importance for the increased fiber formation in Glisson's triads (BECKER, 1971). In short, the resulting pattern can only in a few favor-able cases be distinguished from long-lasting true primary inflammatory lesions, especially from chronic hepatitis. Such favorable conditions exist where the initially finely textured sclerosis within the lobular centers persists for a comparatively long time. This is a typical, or even obligatory event of all of those toxic injuries which proceed without massive cell destruction, as is the case in most of the chronic alcohol intoxications. Finally, one should keep in mind that on the other hand extensive scars ensue within parenchyma in those areas in which many cells have undergone necrosis (see SCHAFFNER, 1971), but which could not be restored by regeneration because of the lasting toxic injury (KLINGE, 1969b); this phenomenon can be seen in sclerosing hyaline necrosis (EDMONDSON et al., 1963; v. SEEBACH et al., 1972).

It follows that some of the hepatoses whose etiology remains unknown necessarily take a chronic course and thus lead to cirrhosis. Though this development has so far only been clearly recognized in chronic alcoholism and in some single cases of halothane intoxication (KLATSKIN and KIMBERG, 1969) and is not generally accepted, it yet may be representative of a significant number of cases. Using a variety of hepatotoxic substances, it is already well documented in animal experiments. Morphological evidence fails, however, to determine the actual percentage of chronic intoxications in human liver cirrhoses.

V. Pathogenetic Considerations

Elucidation of the question of how a hepatotoxic action is triggered is, in general, faced with a variety of difficulties. In some cases the route of application or the dosage of a substance may play a role; more frequently, length of exposure will probably determine the manifestation of hepatotoxicity. Sometimes only the combination of unrelated substances will synergistically lead to the toxic effect. It may be assumed that immunological factors will sometimes be found to play a decisive part. The most important contribution, however, seems to come from constitutional or genetic factors. Via enzyme deficiencies, faulty enzymes, inhibition of protein synthesis, accumulation of toxic intermediates or similar effects, they may transform a substance, which by itself might be quite harmless, into a toxic agent. Nothing definite is known about these various mechanisms. The concept that genetically determined reactions play a central role may explain why animal experiments are often of limited value in the study of hepatotoxic substances and their actions. Results so obtained have frequently been contradicted and corrected by later experience of human pathology. Halothane serves as only one example; even though it had been used without complications in numerous experiments in a variety of animal species, it has occasionally been found to cause severe, even lethal hepatic injuries in humans. This means that the special tolerance of the patient will often or even always have to be taken into account, and in many cases, a pathogenetic elucidation will only be possible for each individual.

References

ABRAHAMS, C., WHEATLEY, A., RUBENSTEIN, A. H., STABLES, D.: Hepatocellular lipofuscin after excessive ingestion of analgetics. Lancet **1964 II**, 621–622.

AFFOLTER, H., HARTMANN, G., KAPFHAMMER, V., SCHEIDEGGER, S.: Akute Massennekrose der Leber nach mehrmaliger Halothan-Narkose. Schweiz. med. Wschr. **94**, 396–400 (1964).

ALBOT, G., JEZEQUEL, A.-M.: Les hepatites virales icterigènes. Semaine Hop. Paris **38**, 517–523 (1962).

ALTMANN, H.-W.: Allgemeine morphologische Pathologie des Cytolasma. In: Handbuch der allgemeinen Pathologie, Bd. II, 1, S. 419–612. Berlin—Göttingen—Heidelberg: Springer 1955.

ALTMANN, H.-W.: Der Zellersatz, insbesondere an den parenchymatösen Organen. Verh. dtsch. Ges. Path. 50, 15–51 (1966).

ALTMANN, H.-W.: Die Histologie der akuten Virus-Hepatitis. Tagg. d. Sozialmediziner, Bad Mergentheim 1970.

ALTMANN, H.-W., KLINGE, O.: Drogen-Hepatopathie. Verh. dtsch. Ges. Path. 56, 194–215 (1972).

ALTMANN, H.-W., LOESCHKE, K., SCHENK, K.: Über das Karyogramm der menschlichen Leber unter normalen und pathologischen Bedingungen. Virchows Arch. path. Anat. 341, 85–111 (1966).

ALTMANN, H.-W., OSTERLAND, U.: Über cytoplasmatische Wirbelbildungen in der Leberzelle der Ratte bei chronischer Thioacetamidvergiftung. Beitr. path. Anat. 124, 1–18 (1961).

ARIAS, I. M.: Effects of a plant acid (Icterogenin) and certain anabolic steroids on the hepatic metabolism of bilirubin and sulfobromophtalein (BSP). Ann. N. Y. Acad. Sci. 104, 1014–1025 (1963).

ASBECK, F., JOIST, H., LÖHRS, U.: Lebervenenthrombose und Ovulationshemmer. Med. Klin. 67, 82–85 (1972).

AYD, F. J.: Chlorpromazine: Ten years experience. J. Amer. med. Ass. 184, 51–54 (1963).

BÄSSLER, R.: Zur Pathogenese seltener Blutungen bei Lebercirrhosen mit Pseudolobulus-Nekrosen. Virchows Arch. path. Anat. 334, 118–131 (1961).

BANNASCH, P.: The cytoplasm of hepatocytes during carcinogenesis. Electron- and light-microscopical investigations of the nitrosomorpholine intoxicated rat liver. Berlin—Heidelberg—New York: Springer 1968.

BANNASCH, P., MÜLLER, H.-A.: Lichtmikroskopische Untersuchungen über die Wirkung von N-Nitrosomorpholin auf die Leber von Ratte und Maus. Arzneimittel-Forsch. 14, 805–814 (1964).

BARONE, P., INFERRERA, C., CARROZZA, G.: Pigments in the Dubin-Johnson Syndrome. In: Pigments in pathology, p. 307–325, ed. M. Wolman. New York—London; Academic Press 1969.

BECKER, J. A. Phenylbutazone Hepatitis. Amer. J. Gastroent. 43, 23–29 (1965).

BECKER, K.: Mucopolysaccharide. In: Alkohol und Leber, S. 293–301, Hrsg. W. Gerok, K. Sickinger und H. H. Hennekeuser. Stuttgart—New York: F.-K. Schattauer 1971.

BECKER, V., MOSER, A.: Endophlebitis hepatica obliterans (Budd-Chiari). Punktatuntersuchung. Acta hepato-splenol. (Stuttg.) 14, 129–142 (1967).

BERNEIS, K., STUDER, A.: Vermehrung von Lipofuscin in der Leber als Folge von Phenacetinabusus. Zentrifugation von menschlicher und tierischer Leber im Dichtegradienten. Virchows Arch. path. Anat. 343, 75–80 (1967).

BERNEIS, K., STUDER, A.: Vergleichende Untersuchungen an Lipofuscin verschiedener Genese aus menschlicher und tierischer Leber. Path. et Microbiol. (Basel) 31, 108–116 (1968).

BHAGWAT, A. G., DEODHAR, D.: Experimental hepatic injury. Produced in the rabbit by glucocorticoids. Arch. Path. 85, 346–456 (1968).

BIAVA, C.: Mallory alcoholic hyalin: a heretofore unique lesion of hepatocellular ergastoplasma. Lab. Invest. 13, 301–320 (1964).

BIAVA, C., MUKHLOVA-MONTIEL, M.: Electron microscopic observation on Councilman-like acidophilic bodies and other forms of acidophilic changes in human liver cells. Amer. J. Path. 46, 775–802 (1965).

BLOODWORTH, J. M. B.: Morphologic changes associated with sulfonylurea therapy. Metabolism 12, 287–301 (1963).

BRAS, G., MCLEAN, E.: Toxic factors in veno-occlusive disease. Ann. N. Y. Acad. Sci. 111, 393–396 (1963).

BRUNI, C.: Hyaline degeneration of rat liver cells studied with the electron microscope. Lab. Invest. 9, 209–215 (1960).

BRUNTSCH, K. H., GRUNZE, H., KÖHN, K.: Komplikation einer Schwangerschaft durch eine Endophlebitis hepatica obliterans unter dem Bilde des Budd-Chiari-Syndroms. Geburtsh. u. Frauenheilk. 18, 1337–1346 (1958).

Burns, J. J., Conney, A. H., Koster, R.: Stimulatory effect of chronic drug administration on drug-metabolizing enzymes in liver microsomes. Ann. N. Y. Acad. Sci. **104**, 881–893 (1963).

Cachin, M.: Iatrogener Ikterus. Münch. med. Wschr. **109**, 1962–1970 (1967).

Clarke, D. A., Philips, F. S., Sternberg, S. S., Stock, C. C., Elion, G. D., Hitschings, G. H.: 6-Mercaptopurine: effects in mouse sarcoma 180 and in normal animals. Cancer Res. **13**, 593–604 (1953).

Clubb, A. W., Giles, C.: Budd-Chiari-Syndrome after oral contraceptivas. Brit. med. J. **1968 I**, 252.

Cohen, A. A., Lawrence, S. H.: Combined hypersensitivity. Reaction to sodium para-aminosalicylate and associated antibacterial drug concurrently administered. Ann. intern. Med. **46**, 893–906 (1957).

Cook, G. C., Sherlock, S.: Jaundice and the relation to therapeutic agents. Lancet **1965 I**, 175–179.

Cullberg, G., Lundström, R., Stenram, U.: Jaundice during treatment with an oral contraceptiva, Lyndiol. Brit. med. J. **1965 I**, 695–697.

Dölle, W., Martini, G. A.: Zusammenstellung von Arzneimitteln, die Leberschädigungungen mit und ohne Gelbsucht verursachen können. Acta hepato-splenol. (Stuttg.) **6**, 225–247 (1959); **9**, 74–85 (1962); **11**, 355–367 (1964).

Dölle, W., Martini, G. A.: Leber. In: Krankheiten durch Arzneimittel, S. 255–283. Hrsg. HINTZ. Stuttgart: Thieme 1966.

Doljanski, L., Rosin, A.: Studies on early changes in the liver of rats treated with various toxic agents, with especial reference to the vascular lesions; histology of the rat's liver in urethane poisoning. Amer. J. Path. **20**, 945–959 (1944).

Dontenwill, W., Hilscher, W., Frank, H.: Tierexperimentelle Untersuchungen zur Wirkung hoher Dosen Cortison und ACTH. Klin. Wschr. **33**, 725–726 (1955).

Dooner, H. P., Hoyl, C., Altaga, C., parada, J.: Jaundice and oral contraceptives. Acta hepato-splenol. (Stuttg.) **18**, 84–94 (1971).

Drill, V. A.: Pharmacology of hepatotoxic agents. Ann. N. Y. Acad. Sci. **104**, 858–874 (1963).

Ecker, J. A.: Phenylbutazone hepatitis. Amer. J. Gastroent. **43**, 23–29 (1965).

Edmondson, H. A., Peters R. L.: Diagnostic problems in liver biopsies. In: Pathology annual 1967, p. 213–242, ed. Sh. C. Symmers. London: Butterworths 1967.

Edmondson, H. A., Peters, R. L., Reynolds, T. B., Kuzma, O. T.: Sclerosing hyaline necrosis of liver in the chronic alcoholic; a recognizable clinical syndrome. Ann. intern. Med. **59**, 646–673 (1963).

Engleman, E. P., Krupp, M. A., Rinehart, J. F., Jones, R. F., Gibson, J. R.: Hepatitis following the ingestion of phenylbutazone. J. Amer. med. Ass. **156**, 98–101 (1954).

Ericsson, J. L. E., Orrenius, S., Holm, I.: Alterations in canine liver cells induced by protein deficiency. Exp. molec. Path. **5**, 329–349 (1966).

Fisher, J. H.: Fatal phenylbutazone hepatitis. Canad. med. Ass. J. **83**, 1211–1212 (1960).

Flax, M. H., Tisdale, W. A.: An electron microscopic study of alcoholic hyaline. Amer. J. Path. **44**, 441–454 (1964).

Fraser, T. N.: Multiple toxic effects of phenylbutazone—report of a fatal case. Brit. med. J. **1955 I**, 1318–1320.

Gerhartz, H.: Hepatotoxische Nebenwirkungen unter cytostatischer Therapie. Arzneimittel-Forsch. **11**, 191–194 (1961).

Gilbert, E. F., DaSilva, A. Q., Queen, D. M.: Intrahepatic cholestasis with fatal termination following norethandrolone therapy. J. Amer. med. Ass. **185**, 538–539 (1963).

Goldstein, G.: Sarcoid reaction associated with phenylbutazone hypersensitivity. Ann. intern. Med. **59**, 97 (1963).

Gordon, B. S., Wolf, J., Krause, T., Shai, F.: Peliosis hepatis and cholestasis following administration of norethandrolone. Amer. J. clin. Path. **33**, 156–165 (1960).

Grayson, M. J., Reilly, M. C. T.: Budd-Chiari-Syndrome after oral contraceptives. Brit. med. J. **1968 I**, 512–513.

Haemmerli, U. P.: Jaundice during pregnancy. With special emphasis on recurrent jaundice during pregnancy and its differential diagnosis. Berlin—Heidelberg—New York: Springer 1966.

HAEMMERLI, U. P., WYSS H. I.: Recurrent intrahepatic cholestasis of pregnancy. Report of 6 cases and review of the literature. Medicine (Baltimore) **46**, 289 (1967).

HARMS, D.: Beitrag zur Kenntnis der akuten Schwangerschaftsfettleber. Frankfurt. Z. Path. **76**, 95–101 (1966).

HAUDENSCHILD, Ch.: Experimentelle Vermehrung von Lipofuscin an der Ratte. Path. et Microbiol. (Basel) **33**, 193–214 (1969).

HAUDENSCHILD, Ch., STUDER, A.: Vermehrung von Lipofuscin am Chinesischen Zwerghamster. Path. et Microbiol. (Basel) **37**, 275–279 (1971).

HERBUT, P. A., SCARICACIOTTOLI, T. M.: Diffuse hepatic necrosis caused by sulfadiazine. Arch. Path. **40**, 94–98 (1945).

HEYMER, A.: Die Bedeutung der medikamentösen Behandlung der Lungentuberkulose in neuer Sicht. Internist (Berl.) **3**, 574–585 (1962).

HILL, K., JÜNGST, B.: Therapiebedingte lokale Pseudophlebitis hyalica obliterans und Hepatosklerose bei kindlicher Leukose. Acta hepato-splenol. (Stuttg.) **16**, 297–307 (1969).

HOFMAN, H. Th.: Zur Frage der Gesundheitsgefährdung durch moderne Kunststoffe und ihre Lösungsmittel. Zbl. Arbeitsmed. **11**, 240–247 (1961).

HOSCHEK, R.: Gesundheitsschäden durch Tetrachlorkohlenstoff. Mat. Med. Nordmark **21**, 257–264 (1969).

HURT, P., WEGMANN, T.: Protrahierter Largactilikterus mit Übergang in primäre biliäre Zirrhose. Acta hepato-splenol. (Stuttg.) **8**, 87–95 (1961).

HUTTERER, R., KLION, F. M., WENGRAF, A., SCHAFFNER, F., POPPER, H.: Hepatocellular adaptation and injury, structural and biochemical changes following dieldrin and methyl-butter-yellow. Lab. Invest. **20**, 455–464 (1969).

ISERI, O. A., GOTTLIEB, L. S.: Alcoholic hyaline and megamitochondria as separate and distinct entities in liver disease associated with alcoholism. Gastroenterology **60**, 1027–1035 (1971).

ISHAK, K. G., GRUNZ, P. R.: Hepatoblastoma and hepatocarcinoma in infancy and childhood. Cancer **20**, 396–422 (1967).

KLATSKIN, G.: Toxic and drug-induced hepatitis. In: Diseases of the liver, 2. ed. p. 453–538, Ed. L. Schiff. London: Pitman 1963.

KLATSKIN, G., KIMBERG, D. V.: Recurrent hepatits attributable to halothane sensitization in an anaesthesist. New Engl. J. Med. **280**, 515–522 (1969).

KLINGE, O.: Toxische Hepatose bei Halothan-Narkose. Klin. Wschr. **43**, 1042–1049 (1965).

KLINGE, O.: Formen und Kennzeichen toxischer Hepatosen. Verh. dtsch. Ges. Path. **53**, 298–302 (1969).

KLINGE, O.: Probleme der Leberregeneration. In: H.-A. Kühn und H. Liehr (Hrsg.) Aktuelle Hepatologie, S. 13–22. Stuttgart: Thieme 1969.

KLINGE, O.: Hepatozelluläre Veränderungen im Leberpunktat bei der chronischen Bleivergiftung des Menschen. Acta hepato-splenol. (Stuttg.) **17**, 151–159 (1970).

KLINGE, O.: Intrahepatische Cholestase und hepatozelullärer Alkoholschaden. In: Alkohol und Leber, S. 373–379, Hrsg. W. Gerok. K. Sickinger und H. H. Hennekeuser. Stuttgart—New York: F. K. Schattauer 1971.

KLINGE, O.: Morphologie und Ätiologie Halothaninduzierter Leberschäden. Verh. dtsch. Ges. Path. **56**, 548–554(1972).

KLINGE, O., ALTMANN, H.-W.: Morphologie toxischer Hepatosen. Münch. med. Wschr. **113**, 1529–1539 (1971a).

KLINGE, O., ALTMANN, H.-W.: Punktathistologie toxischer Leberreaktionen. Lebersymposium in Vulpera, 1971 (b). In: H.-A. KÜHN, N. G. MARKOFF u. M. S. MEIER: Aktuelle Hepatologie, S. 8–22. Stuttgart: Thieme 1973.

KLINGE, O., BANNASCH, P.: Zur Vermehrung des glatten endoplasmatischen Retikulum in Hepatocyten menschlicher Leberpunktate. Verh. dtsch. Ges. Path. **52**, 568–573 (1968).

KLITZEN, W., SILNY, J.: Peliosis hepatis after administration of fluoxysmestosteron. Canad. med. Ass. J. **83**, 860 (1960).

KOHN, N., MYERSON, R. M.: Xanthomatous biliary cirrhosis following chlorpromazine. Amer. J. Med. **31**, 665–670 (1961).

KOHN, R. M., MONTES, M.: Hepatic fibrosis following long acting nicotinic acid therapy: a case report. Amer. J. med. Sci. **258**, 94–99 (1969).

Krass, I.: Budd-Chiari-Syndrome after oral contraceptives. Brit. med. J. **1968I**, 708.

Krüskemper, H. L., Noell, G.: Steroidstruktur und Lebertoxicität. Acta endocr. (Kbh) **54**, 73–84 (1967).

Kühn, H. A., Wegener, F., Hahn, J.: Akute Fettleber in der Schwangerschaft mit tödlichem Ausgang. Acta hepato-splenol. (Stuttg.) **14**, 65–80 (1967).

Kunelis, C. T., Peters, J. L., Edmondson, H. A.: Fatty liver of pregnancy and its relationship to tetracycline therapy. Amer. J. Med. **38**, 359–377 (1965).

Kuntz, E., Liehr, H., Pfingst, W.: Toxische Leberschäden durch Äthionamid. Dtsch. med. Wschr. **92**, 1718–1722 (1967).

Larsson-Cohn, U., Stenram, U.: Jaundice during treatment with oral contraceptive agents, report of two cases. J. Amer. med. Ass. **193**, 422–426 (1965).

Lederer, M., Rosenblatt, P.: Death during sulfathiazole therapy. J. Amer. med. Ass. **119**, 8–18 (1942).

Lepper, M. H., Wolfe, C. K., Zimmermann, H. J., Caldwell E. R. Jr., Spies, H. W., Dowling, H. F.: Effect of largedos es of aureomycin on human liver. Arch. intern. Med. **88**, 271 (1951).

Levi, A. J.: Drug hepatitis. In: The liver, p. 165–177, ed. K. E. Read, London: Butterworth 1967.

Lowell, F. C.: Allergic reactions to sulfonamide and antibiotic drugs. Ann. intern. Med. **43**, 333–344 (1955).

Lund, T., Olsen, St.: Idiopathic renal lipofuscinosis. Two cases. Acta path. microbiol. scand., Section A **78**, 414–420 (1970).

Massmann, W.: Die arbeitshygienische Beurteilung des Dimethylformamid. Zbl. Arbeitsmed. **6**, 207–212 (1956).

Mauer, E. F.: Toxic effects of phenylbutazone (Butazolidin). Review of the literature and report of 23re death following its use. New Engl. J. Med. **253**, 404–410 (1955).

Meacham, G. C., Tillotson, F. W., Heinle, R. W.: Liver damage after prolonged urethane therapy. Amer. J. clin. Path. **22**, 22–27 (1952).

Meyers, J. D., Olson, R. E., Lewis, J. H., Moran, T. J.: Xynthomatous biliary cirrhosis following chlorpromazine, with observations indicating over-production of cholesterol, hyperprothrombinemia and the development of portal hypertension. Trans. Ass. Amer. Phycns **70**, 243–261 (1957).

More, R. H., McMillan, G. C., Duff, L. G.: Pathology of sulfonamide allergy in man. Amer. J. Path. **22**, 703–736 (1946).

Moulding, T. S., Goldstein, S.: Hepatotoxicity due to ethioniamide. Amer. Rev. resp. Dis. **86**, 252–255 (1962).

Müller, H.-A.: Die Chromozentren in den Leberzellkernen der Maus unter normalen und pathologischen Bedingungen. Ergebn. allg. Path. path. Anat. **47**, 144–185 (1966).

Nathan, D. A., Meitus, M. L., Capland, L., Lev, M.: Death following phenylbutazone (Butazolidin) therapy-report of a case. Ann. intern. Med. **39**, 1096–1103 (1953).

Nayak, N. C., Sagreiya, K., Ramalingaswami, V.: Indian childhood cirrhosis: The nature and significance of cytoplasmic hyaline of hepatocytes. Arch. Path. **88**, 631–637 (1969).

Niedobitek, F.: Fibrose der Leber bei akuter Leukose im Kindesalter. Z. Gastroent. **6**, 290–298 (1968).

Nissen, R.: Kolloquium über Gefahren des Halothans. Vorträge aus der praktischen Chirurgie, Heft 68. Stuttgart: Thieme 1963.

Norkin, S. A., Campagna-Pinto, D.: Cytoplasmic hyaline inclusions in hepatoma. Arch. Path. **86**, 25–32 (1968).

Nørredam, K.: Chlorpromazine jaundice of long duration. Acta med. scand. **174**, 163–170 (1963).

Oldershausen, H.-F. v.: Zur Pathogenese des Arzneimittelikterus. In: K. Beck Hrsg. S. 242–247. Ikterus. Stuttgart—New York: F. K. Schattauer 1968.

Oldershausen, H.-G. v., Eggstein, M., Dold, U., Knörr, K.: Ikterus bei intrahepatischer Cholestase nach Gaben von antikonzeptionellen Steroiden. Dtsch. med. Wschr. **90**, 1290–1294 (1965).

Orellana-Alcalde, J. M., Dominguez, J. P.: Jaundice and oral contraceptive drugs. Lancet **1966 II**, 1278–1280.

Peters, R. L., Edmondson, H. A., Kunelis, C. T.: Acuty fatty metamorphosis of the liver in pregnancy. J. Amer. med. Ass. **180**, 767 (1962).

PETERS, R. L., EDMONDSON, H. A., MIKKELSEN, W. P., TATTER, D.: Tetracycline-induced fatty liver in non pregnant patients. Report of six cases. Amer. J. Surg. **113**, 622–632 (1967).

PETERS, R. L., EDMONDSON, H. A., REYNOLDS, T. B., MEISTER, J. C., CURPHEY, T. J.: Hepatic necrosis associated with halothane anaesthesia. Amer. J. Med. **47**, 748–764 (1969).

POPPER, H.: Pathologic 1. dings in jaundice associated with iproniazid therapy. J. Amer. med. Ass. **168**, 2235 (1958).

POPPER, H.: Comments, Wilson's disease, birth defects Original article series, vol. 4 Nr. 2, p. 103, ed. D. Bergsma, New York: The National Foundation 1968.

POPPER, H., SCHAFFNER, F.: Drug induced hepatic injury. Ann. intern. Med. **51**, 1230–1252 (1959).

POPPER, H., RUBIN, E., GARDIOL, D., SCHAFFNER, F., PARONETTO, F.: Drug-induced liver disease: penalty for progress. Arch. intern. Med. **115**, 125–136 (1965).

PORTA, E. A., HARTROFT, W. S.: Lipid pigments in relation to aging and dietary factors (lipofuscins). In: Pigments in pathology, p. 190–235. ed. M. Wolman, New York— London: Academic Press 1969.

PORTER, K. R., BRUNI, C.: An electron microscope study of early effects of 3'-Me-DAB on rat liver cells. Cancer Res. **19**, 997–1009 (1959).

REINL, W., URBAN, H.-J.: Erkrankungen durch Dimethylformamid. Int. Arch. Gewerbepath. Gewerbehyg. **21**, 333–346 (1965).

REMMER, H.: Detoxification of drugs in the liver. In: Progress of liver diseases, eds. H. Popper and F. Schaffner, p. 116–133. New York: Grune & Stratton 1965.

REMMER, H.: Die Entgiftungsfunktion der Leber. In: Kühn, H.-A., und H. Liehr Hrsg. Aktuelle Hepatologie, S. 98–108. Stuttgart: Thieme 1969.

REMMER, H., MERKER, H.-J.: Enzyminduktion und Vermehrung von endoplasmatischem Retikulum in der Leberzelle während der Behandlung mit Phenobarbital (Luminal). Klin. Wschr. **41**, 276–283 (1963).

ROBINSON, D. S., SEAKINS, A.: The development in the rat of fatty livers associated with reduced plasma-lipoprotein synthesis. Biochim. biophys. Acta (Amst.) **62**, 163–165 (1962).

ROTHWELL-JACKSON, R. L.: Budd-Chiari-Syndrome after oral contraceptives. Brit. med. J. **1968 I**, 252.

ROUILLER, Ch.: Experimental toxic injury of the liver. In: The liver, II, ed. Ch. Rouiller p. 335. New York: Academic Press 1964.

RUBIN, E., LIEBER, C. S.: Alcohol-induced hepatic injury in non-alcoholic volunteers. New Engl. J. Med. **278**, 869–876 (1968).

SALFELDER, K., SEELKOPF, C., INGLESSIS, G.: Leberbefunde bei der akutan Phosphorvergiftung des Menschen. Zbl. allg. Path. path. Anat. **108**, 524–529 (1966).

SAMIOS, B., POUNGOURAS, P., THEODOSSIOU, A.: "Lipochrome" hepatosis without jaundice. Acta hepato-splenol. (Stuttg.) **12**, 93–98 (1965).

SCHAFFNER, F.: Electron microscopy of acute alcoholic hepatitis. In: Alkohol and the liver, eds. W. Gerok, K. Sickinger and H. H. Hennekeuser, p. 273–279. Stuttgart— New York: F. K. Schattauer 1971.

SCHAFFNER, F., KNIFFEN, J. C.: Electron microscopy as related to hepatotoxity. Ann. N. Y. Acad. Sci. **103**, 847–857 (1963).

SCHAFFNER, H., POPPER, H.: Cholestasis is the result of hypoactive hypertrophic smooth endoplasmic reticulum in the hepatocyte. Lancet **1969 II**, 355–359.

SCHAFFNER, F., POPPER, H., CHESROW, E.: Cholestasis produces by administration of norethandrolone. Amer. J. Med. **26**, 249–254 (1959).

SCHAFFNER, F., SASAKI, H.: Induced cholestasis. Ultrastructural studies on drug. Rev. int. Hépat. **15**, 461–473 (1965).

SCHNABEL, R., LAHL, R.: Leberparenchymnekrosen durch das neue Antiepileptikum Alpha-Acetoxyphenuron. Zbl. allg. Path. path. Anat. **106**, 42–55 (1964).

SCHMID-BIRCHER, M.: Histologische Organveränderungen beim Kaninchen durch hohe Cortisondosen. Beitr. path. Anat. **114**, 136–150 (1954).

SCHULTZ, V. C., ADAMSON, J. F. Jr., WORKMAN, W. W., NORMAN, T. D.: Fatal liver disease after intravenous administration of tetracycline in high dosage. New Engl. J. Med. **269**, 999–1004 (1963).

Seebach, H. B. v., Dietz, R., Hesoun, P.: Zellularpathologische Aspekte der alkoholischen Leberschädigung des Menschen. Ergebn. inn. Med. Kinderheilk. (im Druck).

Seebach, H. B. v., Leube, G., Hesoun, P.: Lebervergiftung bei chronischer Pharmakotherapie und ihre diagnostischen Kriterien in menschlichen Leberpunktaten. Verh. dtsch. Ges. Path. 56, 484–487 (1972)

Shay, H., Sun, D. C. H.: Massive necrosis of the liver following iproniazid. Ann. intern. Med. 49, 1246 (1958).

Sheehan, H. L.: The pathology of acute yellow atrophy and delayed chloroform poisoning. J. Obstet. Gynaec. Brit. Emp. 47, 49–62 (1940).

Sherlock, S.: Jaundice due to drugs. Proc. roy. Soc. Med. 57, 881–886 (1964).

Sherlock, S.: Hepatic reactions to therapeutic agents. Ann. Rev. Pharmacol. 5, 429–446 (1965).

Sherlock, S.: Prediction of hepatotoxicity due to therapeutic agents in man. Medicine (Baltimore) 45, 453–458 (1966).

Sherman, W. B.: Drug allergy. J. Amer. med. Ass. 140, 447–450 (1949).

Sleeper, J. C., Taylor, M. P., Smith, A. G.: Hepatitis due to p-aminosalcyclic acid hypersensitivity. A clinical-pathologic correlation in two fatal cases. Gastroenterology 39, 208–214 (1960).

Smetana, H. F.: The histopathology of drug-induced liver disease. Ann. N.Y. Acad. Sci. 104, 821–846 (1963).

Smetana, H. F., Hadley, G. G., Sirat, S. M.: Infantile cirrhose: an analytic review of the literature and a report of 50 cases. Pediatrics 28, 107–127 (1971).

Smuckler, E. A.: The ultrastructure of human alcoholic hyaline. Amer. J. clin. Path. 49, 790–797 (1968).

Smuckler, E. A., Arcasoy, M.: Structural and functional changes of the endoplasmic reticulum of hepatic parenchymal cells. Int. Rev. exp. Path. 7, 305–418 (1969).

Speellberg, M. A., Frankel, J. J.: Hepatic and renal damage with azotemia associated iproniazid administration. Amer. J. Gastroent. 37, 64–69 (1962).

Steiner, J. W.: Investigations of allergic liver injury. I. Light, fluorescent and electron microscopic study of the effects of soluble immune aggregates. Amer. J. Path. 38, 411–436 (1961).

Steiner, J. W., Baglio, C. M.: Electron microscopy of the cytoplasm of parenchymal liver cells in naphthyl-isothiocyanate-induced cirrhosis. Lab. Invest. 12, 765–790 (1963).

Stenger, R. J.: Organelle pathology of the liver. The endoplasmic reticulum. Gastroenterology 58, 554–574 (1970).

Studer, A., Schärer, K.: Langfristige Phenacetinbehandlung am Hund mit Berücksichtigung der Leber-Nierenpigmentierung. Schweiz. med. Wschr. 95, 933–941 (1965).

Svoboda, D. J., Higginson, J.: Ultrastructural hepatic changes in rats on a necrogenic diet. Amer. J. Path. 43, 477–495 (1963).

Svoboda, D. J., Manning, R. T.: Chronic alcoholism with fatty metamorphosis of the liver. Mitochondrial alterations in hepatic cells. Amer. J. Path. 44, 645–662 (1964).

Thulin, K. E., Nermark, J.: Seven cases of jaundice in women taking an oral contraceptive, anovlar. Brit. med. J. 1966 I, 584.

Tisdale, W. A.: Focal hepatitis, fever and skin rash following therapy with sulfamethoxypyridazine, a long-acting sulfonamide. New Engl. J. Med. 258, 687–690 (1958).

Torhorst, J., Rohr, H. P., Zollinger, U., Studer, A., Tranzer, J. P.: Ultrastrukturelle Veränderungen der proximalen Tubuluszelle von Rattennieren nach Phenacetinüberlastung. Virchows Arch. path. Anat. 342, 70–84 (1967).

Uram, H., Fisher, B., Fisher E. R.: The hepatotoxic effect of nitrogen mustard after direct intraported injection. Cancer (Philad.) 9, 144–147 (1956).

Valdivia-Barriga, V., Fellman, A., Orellana, J.: Generalised hypersensitivity with hepatitis and jaundice after use of penicillin and streptomycin. Gastroenterology 45, 114–117 (1963).

Walker, C. O., Combes, B.: Biliary cirrhosis induced by chlorpromazine. Gastroenterology 51, 631 (1966).

Wilson, J. W., Leduc, E. H.: Mitochondrial changes in the liver of essential fatty acid deficient mice. J. Cell. Biol. 16, 281–296 (1963).

Yanoff, M., Rawson, A. J.: Peliosis hepatis. Arch. Path. 77, 159–165 (1964).

Institute of Pathology, University of Hamburg, Germany
(Director: Prof. Dr. G. Seifert)

Age-Related Bone Changes*

Histomorphometric Investigation of the Structure of Human Cancellous Bone

GÜNTER DELLING

With 15 Figures

Contents

I. Introduction

Changes in skeleton structure and mass are more striking than in any other organ of the human body during life as a result of extra- and intracellular ageing processes (KORENCHEVSKY, 1961; NORDIN, 1961; ATKINSON and WOODHEAD, 1968; ADAMS et al., 1970, 1971; FRANKS, 1972; HALL, 1972).

* Supported by Deutsche Forschungsgemeinschaft

These changes are also due to exogeneous factors like pressure and tension strength (Pauwels, 1954, 1965) and many other endogenous factors. Physical exercise (Trotter et al., 1960; Saville and Whyte, 1969; Doyle et al., 1970; Dambacher et al., 1971) and different static loads (Motta, 1968) may cause or correct deformities of some skeletal parts. Besides these mechanical functions the bone tissue plays a major role in storage and mobilization of cations and anions. Most important is the regulation of calcium and phosphate homeostasis (Urist and McLean, 1963; Gudmunsson and Woodhouse, 1971). The regulation of other bivalent cations such as magnesium, copper, zinc and cadmium is of equal importance. Due to this high content of stored anions, especially phosphates, the skeleton plays a significant role in the acid-base balance (Barzel, 1969; Wills, 1970; Delling and Donath, 1973). These reactions are directed by hormones and electrolytes which regulate bone cell activity. Any disturbance of these regulating systems leads to changes in cell function (Skosey, 1970). The consequence of these changes is either an increased or decreased bone turnover, resulting in bone structure remodeling and loss or gain of bone mass (Amtmann und Schmitt, 1968).

During human life many endogenous, especially, hormonal factors, show physiological alterations (Sizonenko et al., 1970; Burr et al., 1970; Gryfe et al., 1971), so that a characteristic structure of bone tissue is related to age. The primary aspect is more pronounced at a more advanced age (Garn et al., 1967; Saville, 1965; Bollet, 1968). Pommer (1885, 1925) first described osteoporosis in contrast to rickets as a reduction of bone mass. Since then many investigations have been carried out concerning chemical and physical properties as well as morphological structure of bone (Chalmers and Weaven 1966; Mueller et al., 1966; Krokowski, 1966; Weber et al., 1969; West and Reed, 1970). Special attention has been paid to the differentiation of age-related bone mass reduction and the pathological phenomenon of osteoporosis (Arnold et al., 1966; Newton and Morgan, 1968; Atkinson et al., 1962; Albanese et al., 1969; Currey, 1969; Arman and Reizenstein, 1971; Exton-Smith et al., 1971; Börner et al., 1972; Boukhris and Becker, 1972). The clinical-diagnostic application of these experiences was very difficult because of many technical problems and great variations of physiological data (Bauer et al., 1958). The development and use of quantitative histological methods (Ball, 1957; Henning, 1956, 1958; Frost, 1963; Nordin, 1964; Jowsey et al., 1965; Müller und Schenk, 1966; Merz, 1967; Woods et al., 1968; Wu et al., 1970; Bordier and Tun Chot, 1972) showed new possibilities for clarifying the pathogenesis of bone disease. For this purpose the knowledge of the physiological structure of bone in healthy subjects during human life is fundamental. The early diagnosis of a metabolic osteopathy, for instance, in primary hyperparathyroidism or in chronic renal failure, may have considerable consequences for the prognosis of the disease (Dambacher et al., 1972b).

In generalized osteopathy a biopsy of any part of the skeleton can be taken with the idea that this tissue is representative for the whole skeleton. Today

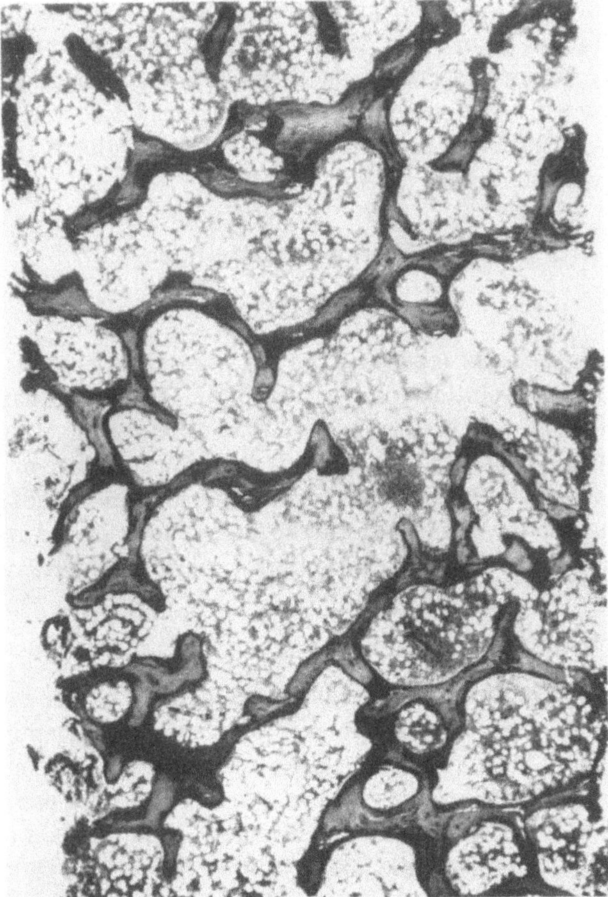

Fig. 1. Low magnification of an iliac crest biopsy (renal osteopathy). The architecture of
cancellous bone is well preserved. Goldner stain. 10 ×

the usual method is the biopsy of the iliac crest. In addition, it is possible to
take biopsies of localized bone processes and to investigate large tissue samples
(whole iliac crest, vertebrae etc.) of necropsies.

II. Modern Techniques for Investigation of Bone Tissue
1. Iliac Crest Biopsy

Most important for obtaining sufficient material is the biopsy technique
(SACKER and NORDIN,1954; BARTELHEIMER und SCHMITT-ROHDE,1957; BARTEL-
HEIMER, 1963; BECK and NORDIN, 1960; WILLIAMS and NICHOLSON, 1963;
LOZANO-TONKIN,1968). The method described by BURKHARDT (1966) has proved
to be an optimal procedure. About 5 cm posterior to the anterior superior iliac
spine a bone cylinder of 20 mm length and 4 mm in diameter is extracted with
an electrical boring machine under local anesthesia after incision of the skin

and the periosteum (Fig. 1). BORDIER and TUN CHOT (1972) prefer the trans-iliacal biopsy about 7 cm below the iliac crest. By using this method one gets only a short biopsy cylinder with cancellous bone, because at a more advanced age the os ilium may be very thin in this region. Of course, no diagnosis is possible when insufficient material is available, for instance, only cortical bone and periosteum.

2. Histological Methods

a) Fixation

According to SCHENK (1965) and in our own experience (DELLING, 1972), fixation in Carnoy's solution (60 parts absolute ethanol, 30 parts chloroform, 10 parts acetic acid) for three hours results in an excellent preservation of the tissue. One can also use 70 % ethanol, but then the structure of bone and bone marrow cells is less well preserved. Fixation in formalin yields unsatisfactory results. Storage of the tissue in formalin over a long period results in decalcification and in the simultaneous dissolving of performed tetracycline labelling.

b) Methylmethacrylate Embedding and Cutting Procedure

Only after preparing an undecalcified specimen of bone tissue can one make a statement concerning the real structure of mineralized bone, the osteoid seams and their relation to bone cells. For this reason the biopsy or autopsy material must be embedded in a material which has the same physical qualities of bone but which in addition cuts well (HIRSCH and BOELLARD, 1958; EGER et al., 1964; SCHENK, 1965; JOWSEY et al., 1965; BURKHARDT, 1966; SHIMO, 1968; MAGILL and GUNNING, 1968; ZAMBERLAND et al., 1969; GREEN, 1970; DELLING, 1972). Sections of 1–10 µ thickness can be prepared from bone specimen embedded in methylmethacrylate. Furthermore it is possible to use the remaining material for ground sections (20–200 µ), which may be necessary for special problems, for instance, the degree of mineralization of the periosteocytic matrix and of the other bone tissue (HEUCK, 1970). Undecalcified sections today are usually stained according to GOLDNER's method (GOLDNER, 1938). The bone sections thus stained allow a clear demarcation of the osteoid seams from the mineralized bone. The osteoblasts as well as the osteoclasts can easily be distinguished by their intense orange color.

III. Histological Structure of Bone (after Undecalcified Preparation)

1. Osteoblasts and Osteoid Seams

The osteoblasts form the osteoid seams — the nonmineralized bone matrix (HERRING, 1968; HALL, 1971). These cells originate from the so-called pro-

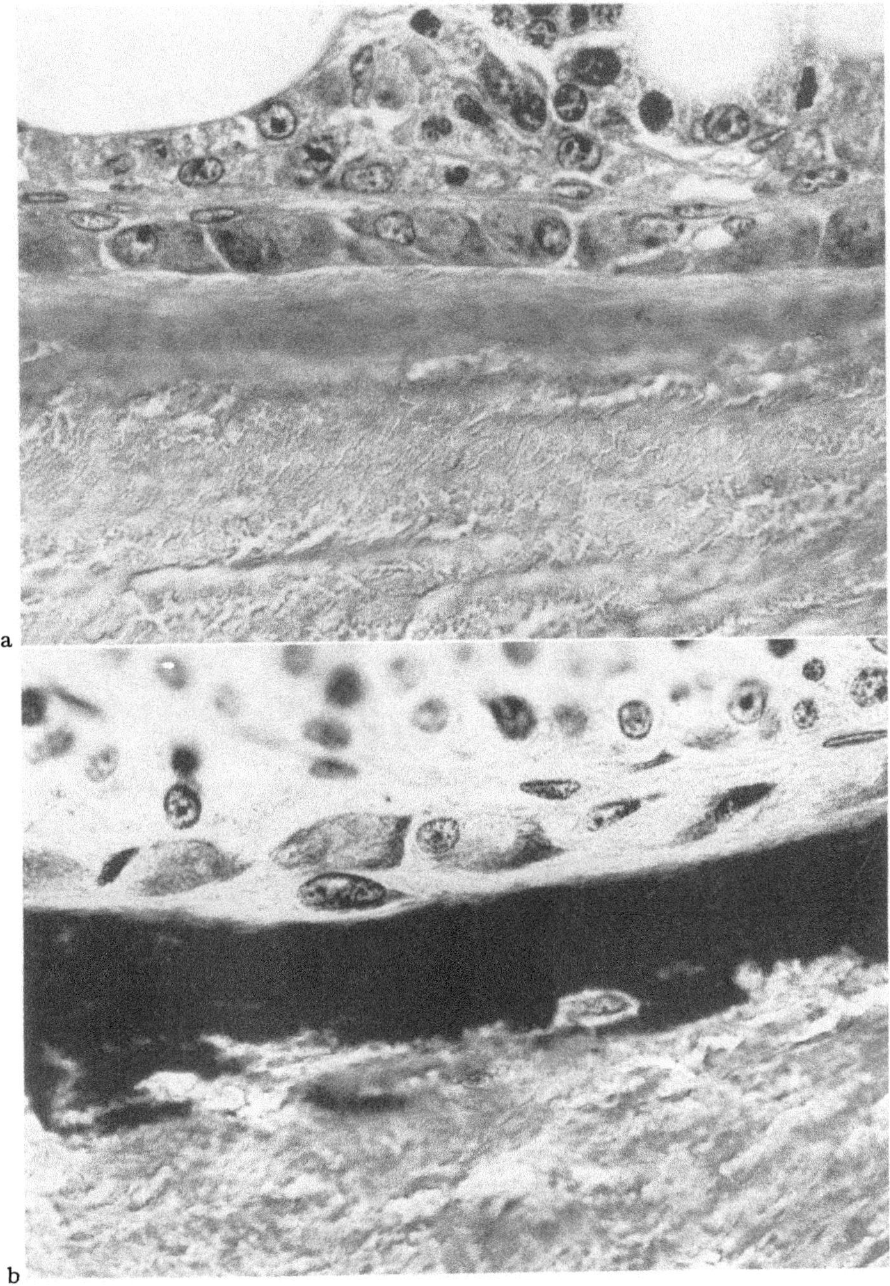

Fig. 2a–c. Active osteoblasts covering broad osteoid seams. a, Giemsa stain, 800×.
b and c, Goldner stain, 800 × and 600 ×

genitor cells. In contrast to fibroblasts which form collagen tissue all around
themselves, the osteoblasts secrete the collagen precursors and ground substances (SCHUBERT and PRAS, 1968) in one direction only (FROST, 1966). In

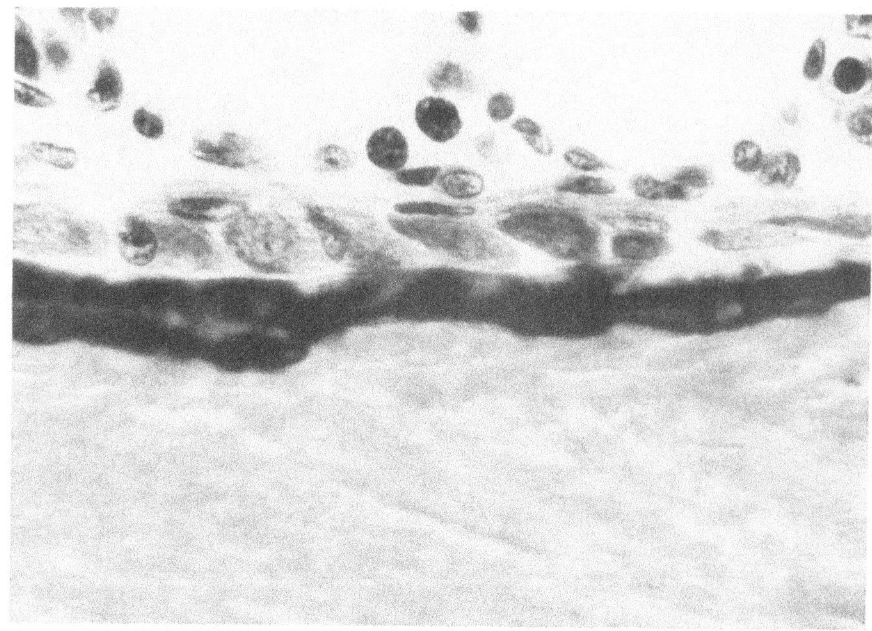

Fig. 2c

this way a special and directed architecture develops. Precursors of collagen are sythesized within the osteoblasts and secreted throughout the cell membrane. On the outside, the cell's collagen polymerizes with ground substances to the osteoid seams. A continously increasing concentration of calcium exists from the osteoid near the marrow space to the mineralized bone. Along the mineralization border, hydroxyapatite is formed. The average thickness of the osteoid seam is 12 μ. Since osteoblasts produce about 1–2 μ of seam thickness per day, the conversion of one seam to mineralized bone takes about 8–9 days (FROST, 1968, 1969). Regarding the morphological function of the osteoblasts, two types of osteoid can be distinguished. One form of osteoid is covered by large, active osteoblasts (Fig. 2). These cells regulate or at least influence the mineralization of the osteoid seams just produced (primary mineralization). The second form of osteoid is covered by flat, inactive osteoblasts (resting cells)—so-called inactive seams. Here the mineralization occurs independently from the bone cells (secondary mineralization). The mineralization can be demonstrated (Fig. 3) by means of tetracycline labelling (KIENITZ, 1965; FROST, 1968, 1969; MUENZENBERG and GEBHARDT, 1970).

2. Osteoclasts and Howship's Lacunae

The oldest parts of mineralized bone were resorbed by polynucleated osteoclasts. The lacunae of Howship of different depths are the result of this process (Fig. 4). The half-life of the osteoclasts is very short, and after com-

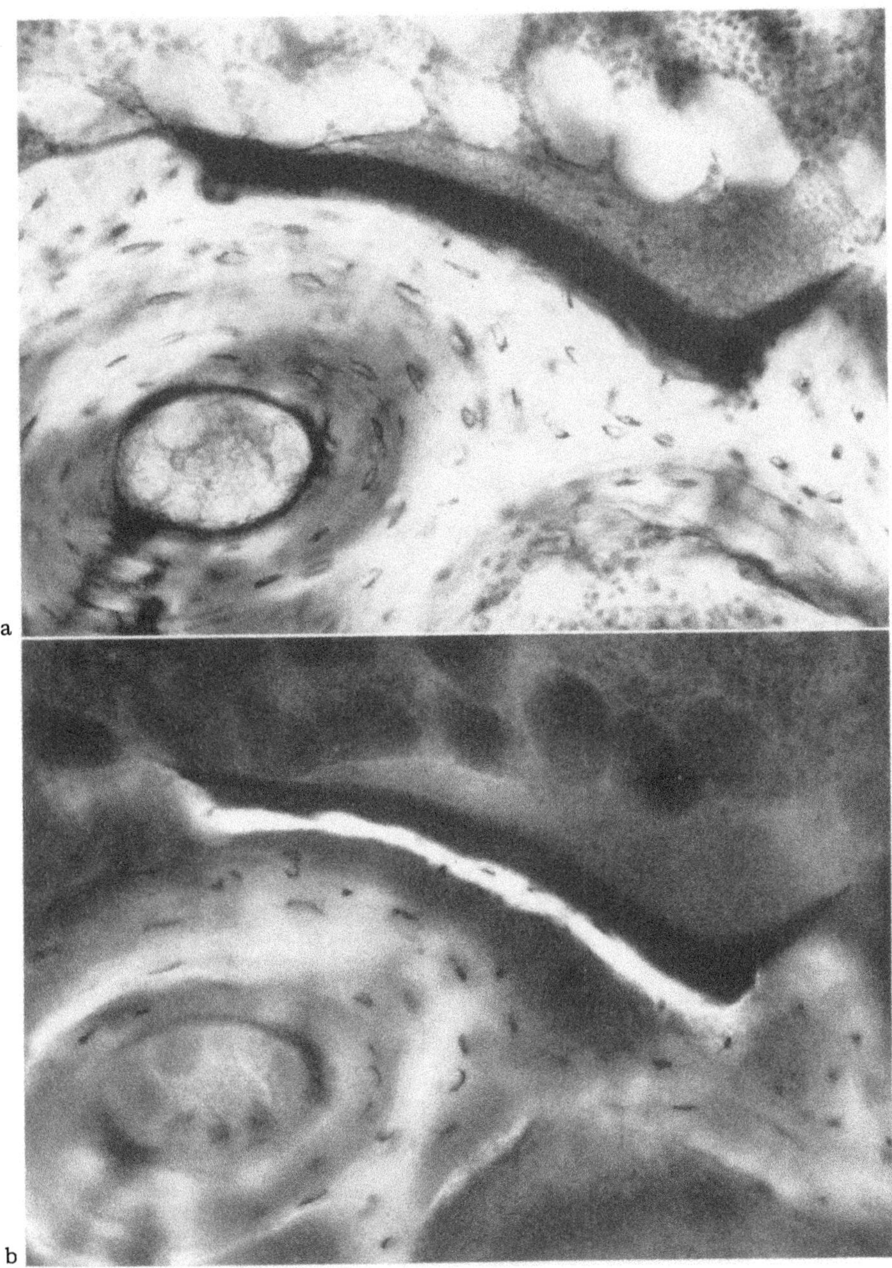

Fig 3a–c. Tetracycline labelling. a 100 μ thick ground section of cancellous bone. In black color an osteoid seam. Basic fuchsin block staining, 200×. b Same region in ultraviolet light. Intensive (yellow) fluorescence at the mineralization border between osteoid and mineralized bone. c 10 μ thick section in ultraviolet light. On the right primary mineralization, on the left secondary mineralization without osteoblasts. Unstained, 100×

pleted resorption an empty lacuna remains; thus, empty lacunae are the expression of an earlier state of resorption and not an actual process. Under the electron microscope osteoclasts have a ruffled border at the bone site

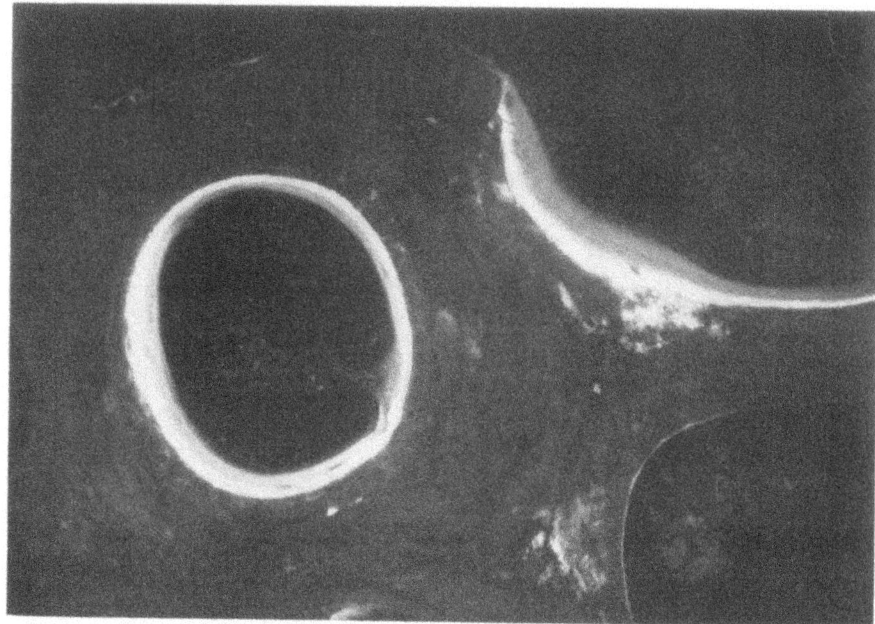

Fig. 3c

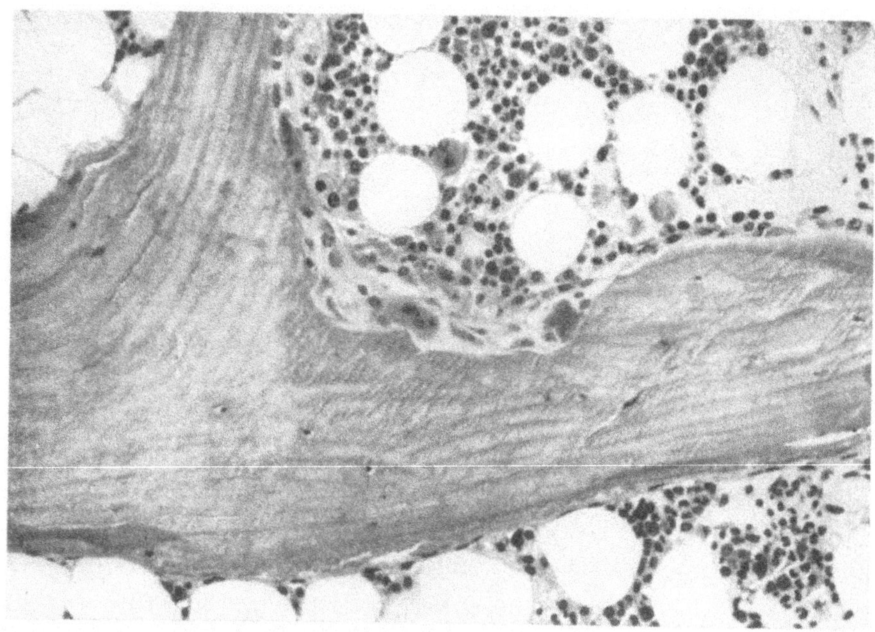

a

Fig. 4a–c. Feature of osteoclastic resorption. a: Three large osteoclasts in a Howship's lacuna, Goldner stain, 180×. b and c: Small osteolcasts in flat resorption lacunae. Goldner stain, 460×

which contains a large amount of acid phosphatase. Moreover, the cytoplasm contains a great number of cell organelles which correspond to a high cell activity.

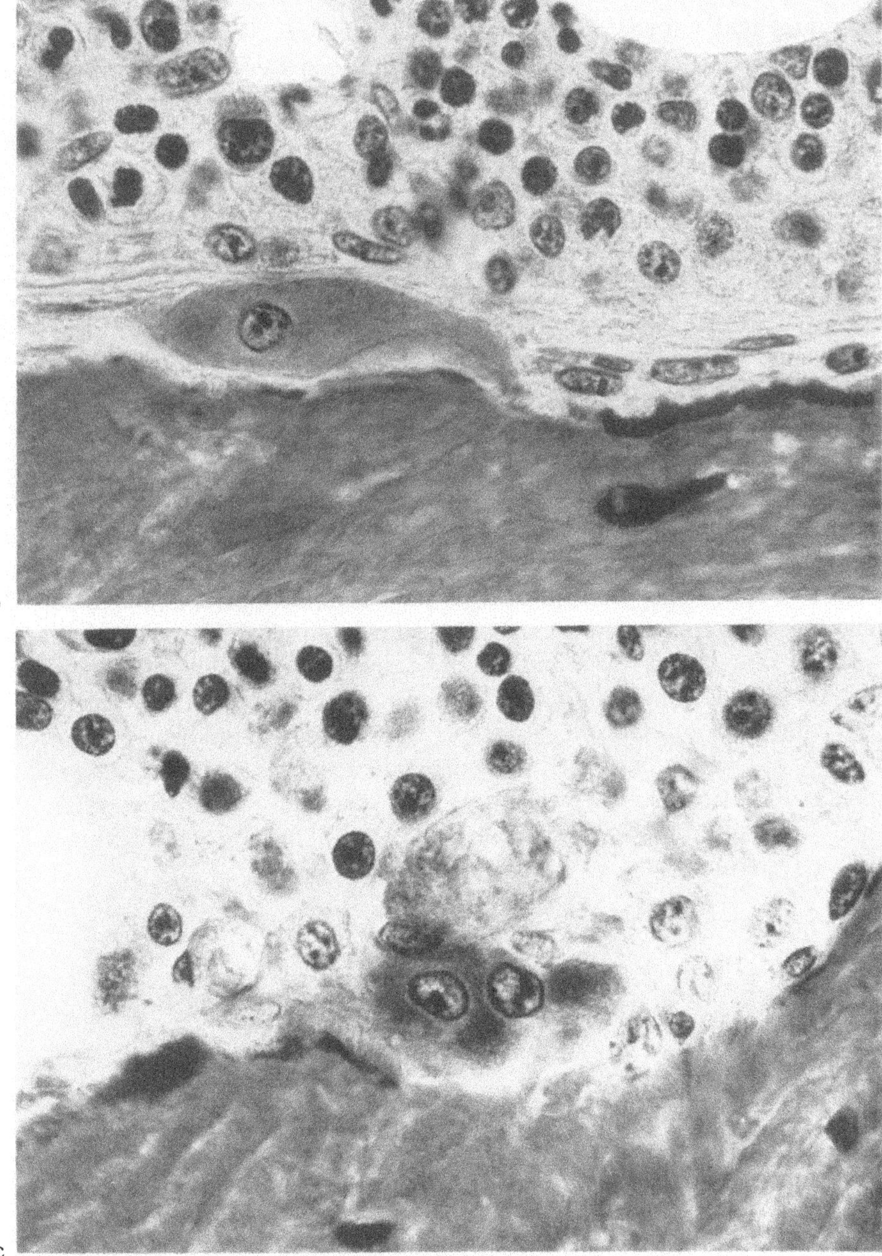

Fig. 4 b and c

3. Inactive Surface of Cancellous Bone

The main part of the cancellous bone surface is, however, under physio-logical conditons inactive, which means that neither osteoid seams nor How-ship's lacunae cover it. This so-called neutral surface borders on the marrow space. It is still not known whether the surface is completely or incompletely covered by mesenchymal cells. These very flat cells remain connected with the processes of the osteocytes. TALMAGE (1970) supposed this group of cells to play an important role in the regulation of serum calcium and phosphorus.

4. Osteocytes and Pericellular Matrix

The osteoblast after being surrounded by organic matrix becomes an osteocyte. By means of electron microscopy the characteristic stages in ageing of bone can be seen in the osteocytes (BAUD, 1962, 1968; JANDE, 1971). Osteoblastic as well as osteoclastic activity of the osteocytes may occur (Figs. 5 and 6). The main role of this cell group is to carry the calcium from the bone to the extracellular fluid and vice versa (BELANGER, 1969; TALMAGE, 1970). Regulation of the mineral and water content of bone by osteocytes results in optimal mechanical properties (FROST, 1968). The high metabolic activity of an osteocyte is made possible by the processes of all osteocytes being connected with each other. The processes connect osteoblasts and osteoclasts as well. The surface of the surrounding matrix—the lacuna wall—consists of $20 \text{ mm}^2/\text{mm}^3$ bone, and $200 \text{ mm}^2/\text{mm}^3$ bone for the surface of the canaliculae containing the cell processes (MÜLLER and SCHENK, 1966). The wall of the lacuna consists of collagen fibers and ground substance as well as of mineralized bone. In some lacunae walls a membrane can be detected by electron microscopy, the function and importance of which is still unknown (DONATH and DELLING, 1971; SCHERFT, 1972). Hydroxyapatite crystals cover the collagen fibers so that an optimal mechanical structure and a metabolic system are formed (PAUWELS, 1954, 1965; ROBINSON and ELLIOTT, 1957; KNEESE, 1958, 1963; GLIMCHER, 1968).

IV. Quantitative Analysis of the Volume and Surfaces of Cancellous Bone

1. Methods

DELESSE described in 1866 the basic idea of the morphometric technique which is still used today. He suggested that in a histologic section, one can determine the volume from the area of an unknown body, and the surface, from the length of the circumference. Many different methods are used to obtain these measurements. HENNING (1956, 1958) developed the so-called point counting method ("hit method") which allows the determination of the volume and of the surfaces by means of points and parallel lines. MERZ (1967) described a new grid, which is independent of the direction of the measured structure and of the angle between the lines and the surfaces. He used parallel wave lines with a raster of 36 points. This system reduces the time of measurement to a minimum.

The special grid is in the eyepiece of the microscope. The distance between two points should be approximately equal to the diameter of the trabecula.

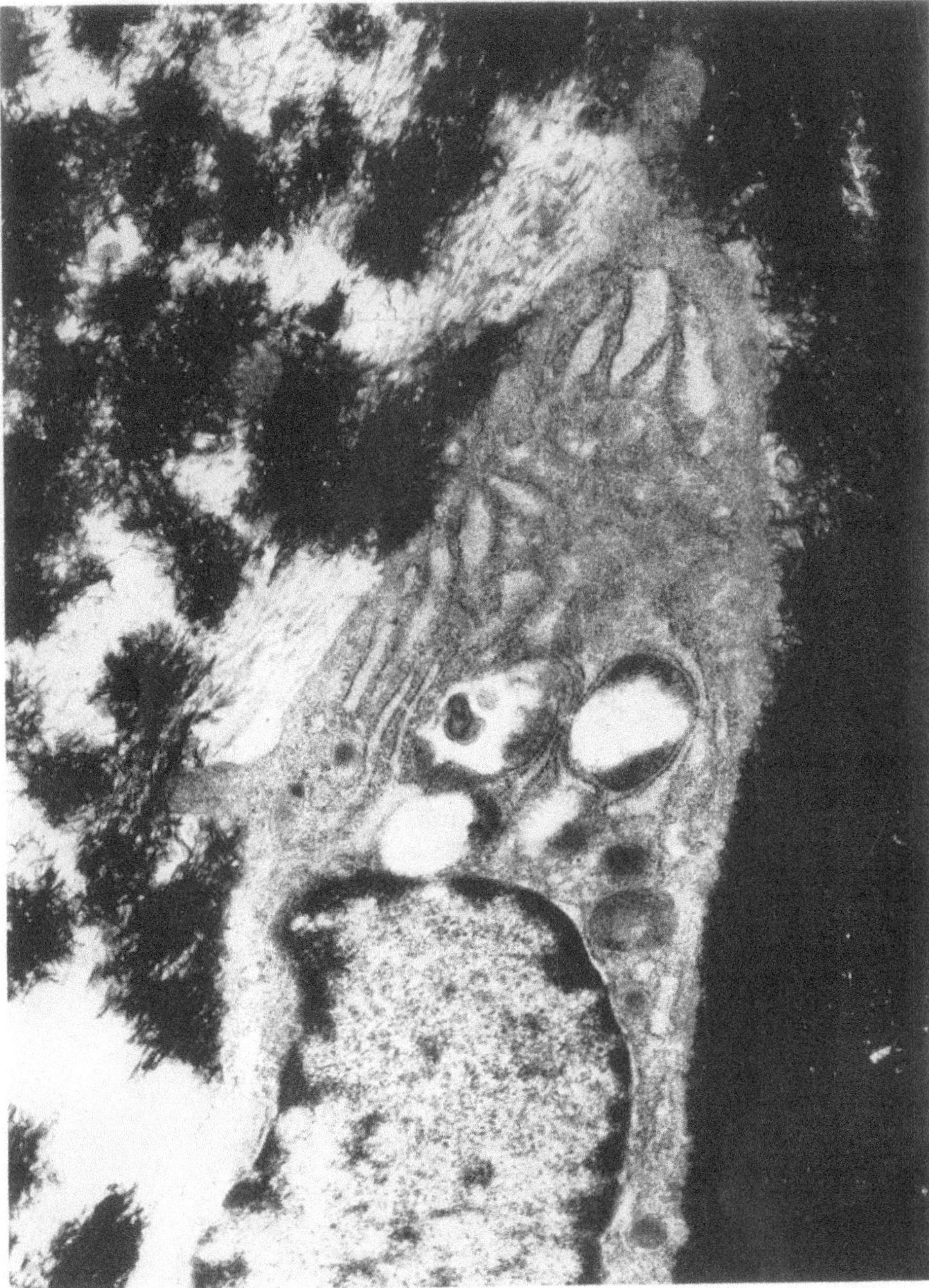

Fig. 5. Ultrastructure of a young osteocyte with many crystallization centers in the surrounding matrix. 18 500 ×

The absolute distance between the two points (grid constant) is determined with the usual object micrometer. The most serviceable magnification lies between 120 and 250. The hits on the mineralized bone and osteoid seams

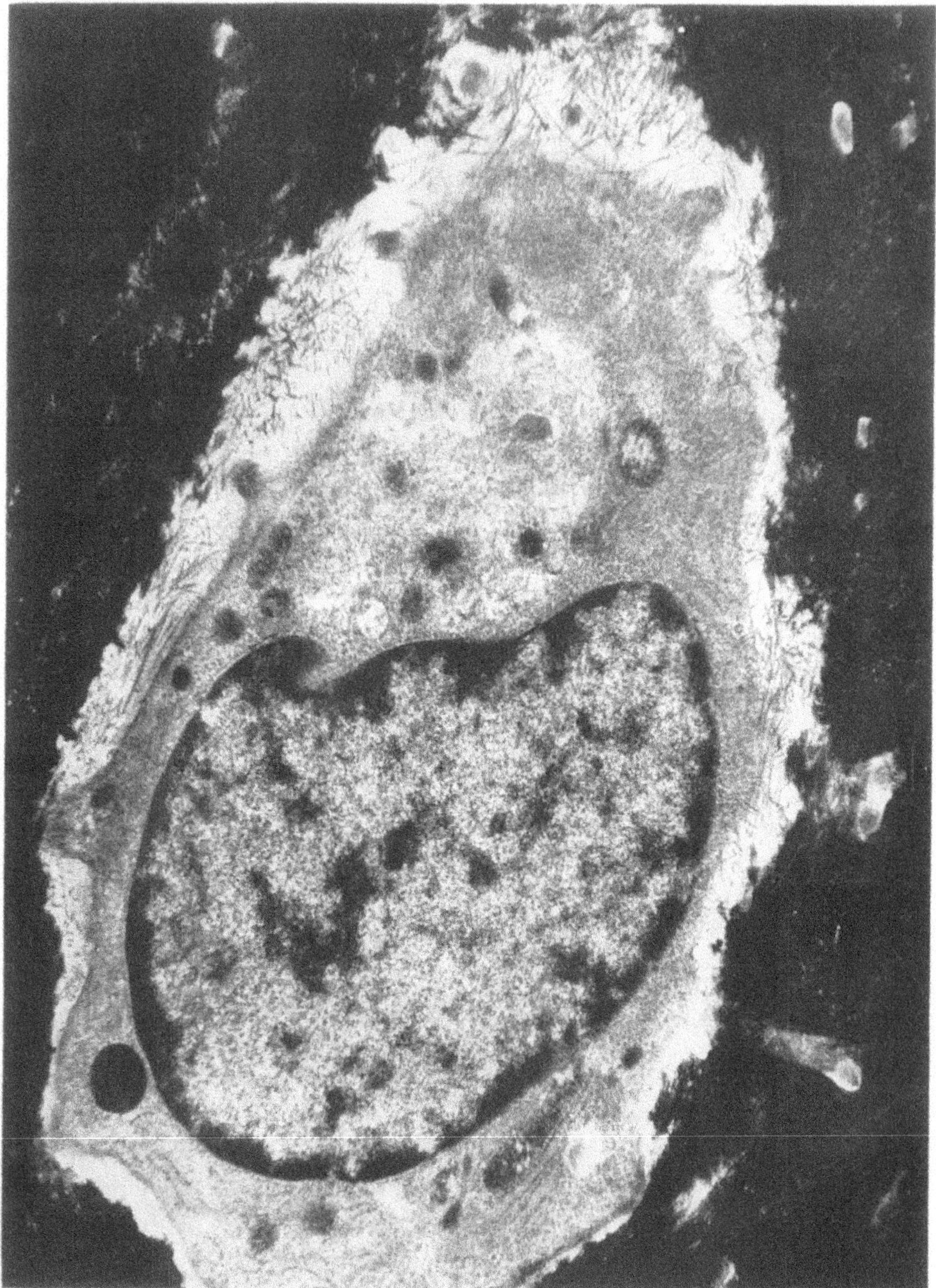

Fig. 6. Ultrastructure of a large, inactive (?) osteocyte. Many processes and canaliculi within the mineralized bone. 8 500 ×

were estimated as well as the intersections between the trabecular surface and the wave lines. In this way the osteoid with and without osteoblasts as well as lacunae with and without osteoclasts are differentiated. The inactive surface can be determined by substraction of these "hits" from the total number of intersections. The number of osteoclasts of each measured field is counted in addition. The measurement should cover 30–40 mm². The following parameters can be calculated when the first listed data are known:

F = number of measured fields
P = hits on mineralized bone and osteoid seams
P_o = hits on nonmineralized bone (osteoid seams)
N = total number of intersections
N_{ob} = intersections of osteoid seams with osteoblasts
N_{io} = intersections of osteoid seams without osteoblasts
N_{ho} = intersections of Howship's lacunae with osteoclasts
N_{he} = intersections of empty Howship's lacunae
N_{ocl} = number of osteoclasts of all measured fields

2. Parameters of the Volume and Structure of Cancellous Bone

a) Volumetric Density (V_v)

$$V_v = \frac{P \times 100}{F \times 36} \; (\%).$$

Percentage of the bone volume (mineralized and nonmineralized) in a unit volume of total bone tissue.

b) Surface Density (S_v)

$$S_v = \frac{N}{F} \times k_{sv} \quad (k_{sv} = \frac{4}{\pi \times 36 \times d}) \; mm^2/mm^3.$$

Border surface of trabecular bone with the marrow space per unit volume of total bone tissue.

c) Specific surface (S/V)

$$S/V = \frac{N}{P} \times k_{s/v} \quad (k_{s/v} = \frac{4}{\pi \times d}) \; (mm^2/mm^3).$$

Surface of trabecular bone in relation to a unit volume of trabecular bone (mineralized and nonmineralized substance without the marrow space).

3. Parameters of the Volume and Structure of New Bone Formation

a) Volumetric Density of the Osteoid (Osteoid Volume; V_{vo})

$$V_{vo} = \frac{P_o \times 100}{F \times 36} \; (\%).$$

Percentage of osteoid volume in a unit volume of total bone tissue.

b) Osteoid Seam Thickness ($\overline{S}$)

$$\overline{S} = \frac{V_{vo}}{S_{vvs}} \; (\mu).$$

Thickness of osteoid seams in case of the known volume and absolute extent of total osteoid seams (see below).

c) Surface Extent of Active Seams (OB)

$$OB = \frac{N_{ob}}{N} \times 100 \ (\%).$$

Surface extent of osteoid seams with osteoblasts as percentage of the total trabecular bone surface.

d) Surface Extent of Inactive Seams (IO)

$$IO = \frac{N_{io}}{N} \times 100 \ (\%).$$

Surface extent of osteoid seams without osteoblasts as percentage of the total trabecular bone surface.

e) Total Extent of Osteoid Seams (OS)

$$OS = \frac{N_{ob} + N_{io}}{N} \times 100 \ (\%).$$

Total surface extent of seams with and without osteoblasts as percentage of the total trabecular bone surface.

f) Relative Activity of Osteoblasts (ROBA)

$$ROBA = \frac{N_{ob}}{N_{ob} + N_{io}} \times 100 \ (\%).$$

g) Surface Density of Osteoid Seams (S_{vos})

$$S_{vos} = \frac{S_v \times OS}{100} \ (mm^2/mm^3).$$

Absolute value of the surface of total osteoid seams per unit volume of total bone tissue.

4. Parameters of the Structure of Bone Resorption

a) Surface Extent of Howship's Lacunae with Osteoclasts (HO)

$$HO = \frac{N_{ho}}{N} \times 100 \ (\%).$$

Surface extent of resorption cavities with osteoclasts as percentage of the total trabecular bone surface.

b) Surface Extent of Empty Howship's Lacunae (HE)

$$HE = \frac{N_{he}}{N} \times 100 \ (\%).$$

Surface extent of resorption cavities without osteoclasts as percentage of total trabecular bone surface.

c) Total Surface Extent of Howship's Lacunae (HT)

$$HT = \frac{N_{ho} + N_{he}}{N} \times 100 \ (\%).$$

Extent of the total surface of resorption cavities with and without osteoclasts as percentage of total trabecular bone surface.

d) Relative Osteoclastic Activity (ROCA)

$$\mathrm{ROCA} = \frac{N_{ho}}{N_{ho} + N_{he}} \times 100 \ (\%).$$

Surface extent of lacunae with osteoclasts as percentage of the total extent of Howship's lacunae.

e) Index of Osteoclasts (OI)

$$\mathrm{OI} = \frac{N_{ocl}}{N} \times k_{oi} \ (900 \times \pi \times d).$$

Number of osteoclasts divided by surface density.

f) Surface Density of Total Extent of Howship's Lacunae (S_{vht})

$$S_{vht} = \frac{S_v \times \mathrm{HT}}{100} \ (\mathrm{mm^2/mm^3}).$$

Absolute value of the total extent of Howship's lacunae per unit volume of total bone tissue.

5. Parameters of the Structure of Inactive Bone Surface

a) Extent of Inactive Trabecular Bone Surface (IS)

$$\mathrm{IS} = \frac{N - (N_{cb} + N_{io} + N_{ho} + N_{he})}{N} \times 100 \ (\%).$$

Inactive, or neutral trabecular bone surface as percentage of the total trabecular bone surface.

b) Surface Density of Inactive Surface (S_{vis})

$$S_{vis} = \frac{S_v \times \mathrm{IS}}{100} \ (\mathrm{mm^2/mm^3}).$$

Absolute value of the extent of inactive trabecular bone surface per unit volume of total bone tissue.

V. Age-Related Changes of the Volumes and Surfaces of Human Cancellous Bone

Many factors influence the structure of the cancellous bone. Static and hormonal influences (NORDIN, 1966; NORDIN et al., 1966; KUHLENKORDT et al., 1966; NILSSON, 1969), changes of blood supply (HRUZA and WACHTLOVA, 1969; ROCKOFF et al., 1969) and of the electrical potentials of the apatite crystals might be the result of an increased or decreased bone turnover. A survey of the macroscopic structure at different stages of human age is shown in Figs. 8 and 9. The normal as well as the pathological features of the bone structure are formed by four essential processes (formation, mineralization, resorption, osteocytic activity) of bone turnover, shown in Fig. 7. The following sections contain the physiological changes of the cancellous bone of the iliac crest from birth to 90 years of age.

9*

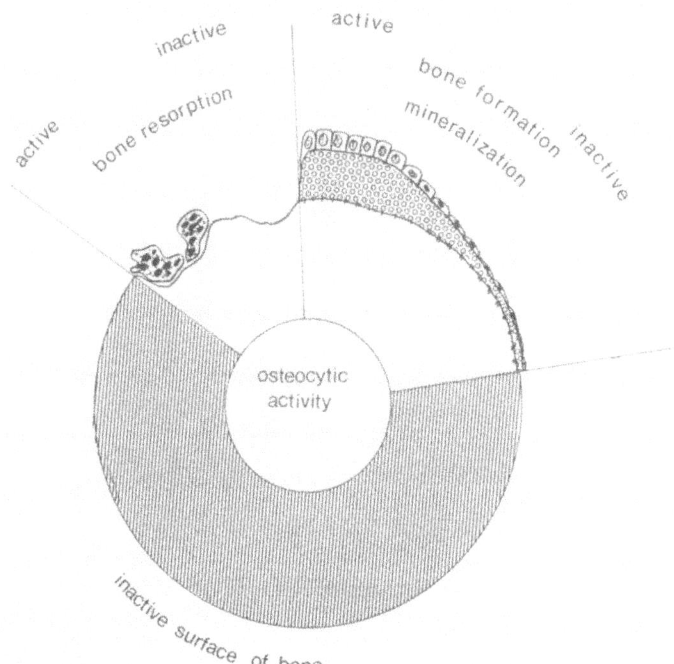

Fig. 7. Schematic presentation of the four important processes which influence the bone structure. Bone resorption by polynucleated osteoclasts resulting in an empty lacuna. The empty lacuna is repaired by active osteoblasts and osteoid. Here the primary mineralization takes place. Osteoid seams without osteoblasts disappear more slowly than the active seams. The main part of cancellous bone is inactive. The inner surfaces are the result of the osteocytic activity

1. Changes in the Structure of Cancellous Bone

a) Volumetric Density (V_v)

The total bone tissue (bone and marrow space) contains about 20% cancellous bone (Fig. 10). The remaining 80% consists of bone marrow, fat cells and blood vessels (Jowsey, 1960; Frost, 1963; Sissons, 1964; Nordin, 1964; Garner and Ball, 1966; Barer and Jowsey, 1967; Wakamatsy and Sissons, 1969; Schenk and Merz, 1969; Olah and Schenk, 1969; Kuhlenkordt, 1970; Merz and Schenk, 1970a; Ellis and Peart, 1972; Delling, 1973). In newborns the value is appreciably higher — up to 40% of the total bone tissue is trabecular bone. This trabecular bone is in part lamellar, in part fibrous in structure. At the end of puberty a reduction to 20% occurs. This value remains nearly constant up to the 5th decade of life. From here a gradual loss of bone mass takes place in the ensuing years (Dequeker, 1972). After mazeration of the bone, the loss of mass can easily be detected by the naked eye (Figs. 8 and 9; Vost, 1963; Wagner, 1965; Urist et al., 1970; Vitalli, 1970). The cancellous bone is initially structured on an undirected lamina system. After dissolution of the laminas, the main trajectorial architecture of

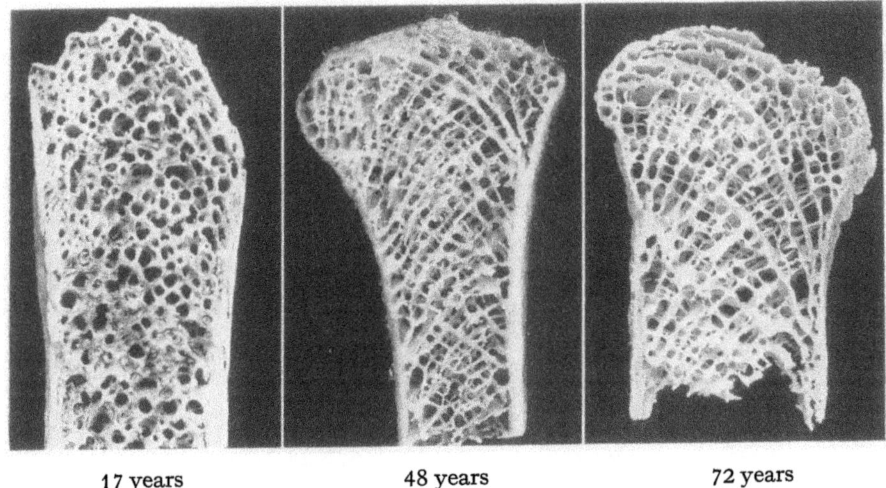

Fig. 8. Iliac crest specimen after mazeration by 10% KOH (3 hours). From left to right: 17 years, 48 years, 72 years. 3 ×

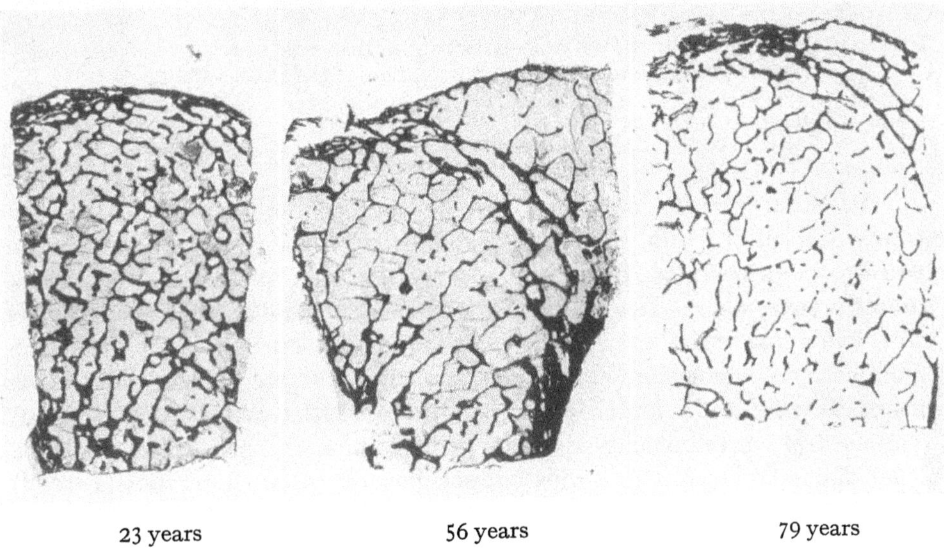

Fig. 9. Sections of the iliac crest at low magnification. From left to right: 23 years, 56 years, 79 years. Note the reduction of bone mass and compensated hypertrophy at an advanced age. Kossa modification (Krutsay). 2.5 ×

the bone tissue appears. The rarefaction of bone, which starts in the central part of the iliac crest results in greater marrow spaces with fat tissue and islets of blood marrow (Fig. 9). For this reason iliac crest biopsies of insufficient length may not show the whole process of rarefaction in early stages. This demonstrates that the diagnosis of the beginning of osteoporosis is not possible by the determination of the volumetric density alone. In advanced stages of osteoporosis, however, the volumetric density is remarkably decreased when compared with normal cases. Eger *et al.* (1967), Dunnill *et al.* (1967), Bell *et al.* (1967), Atkinson (1967), Popowitz and Johnston (1971), and Dequeker *et al.* (1971) found similar results for the cancellous bone of the femur head and of the vertebrae.

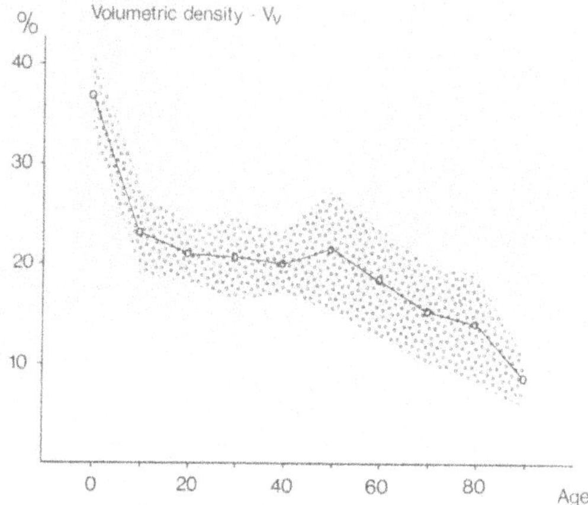

Fig. 10. Volumetric density of the cancellous bone of iliac crest in relation to age. Shaded area indicates the standard deviation of the mean value

b) Specific Surface (S/V)

The surface of the cancellous bone depends on the diameter of the bone trabeculae, on the total bone mass (volumetric density) and on the surface pattern. Eger *et al.* (1967) investigated the diameter of the bone trabecula—its reciprocal value is the specific surface (S/V). It shows a gradual increase with increasing age as a result of compensated hypertrophy. The total bone mass becomes smaller but some trajectoral lines become broader due to local increased new bone formation (Eger, 1965; Merz and Schenk, 1970a). This contrary development—decrease of bone mass and increase of the trabecular diameter—results in a constant specific surface in all decades (Table 1). Only with the development of an osteoporosis does the specific surface increase because compensated hypertrophy is lacking. That means the trabecular diameter of the bone is in fact less (Eger, 1965; Schenk and Merz, 1969; Merz and Schenk, 1970a, b; Kuhlenkordt, 1970; Vitalli, 1970).

c) Surface Density (S_v)

The surface density expresses the total surface of cancellous bone per unit volume of total bone tissue. It is about 4 mm² per mm³ total bone tissue during the first two decades and decreases after this period to 2 mm²/mm³ in the more advanced age groups (Table 1). In the case of an increased resorption especially within the trabecular bone, the surface density increases. In primary and secondary hyperparathyroidism the surface density rises to 6 or 7 mm²/mm³ (Binswanger *et al.*, 1971; Delling, 1972).

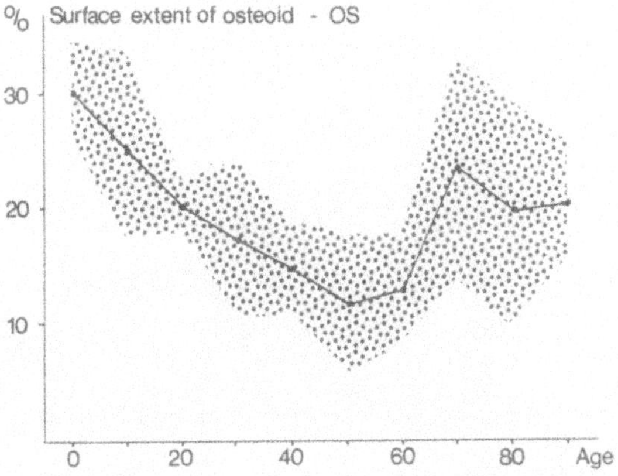

Fig. 11. Total surface extent of osteoid seams as a percentage of total bone surface. The shaded area represents the standard deviation

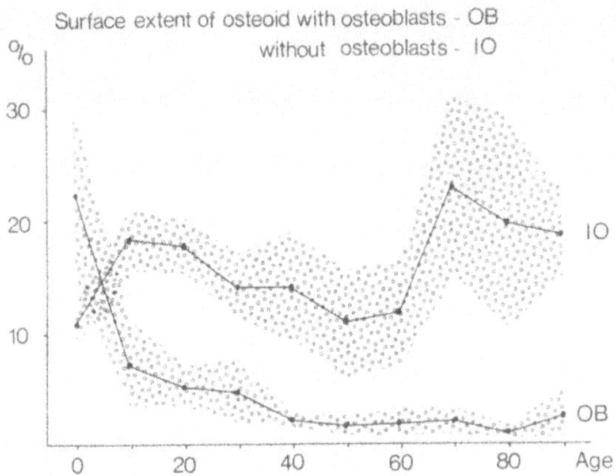

Fig. 12. Surface extent of osteoid seams with and without osteoblasts. Note the decrease of osteoid with osteoblasts after the 3rd and 4th decade. The shaded areas indicate the standard deviation

2. Changes in the New Bone Formation

a) Volumetric Density of the Osteoid (V_{v^o})

The volumetric density of osteoid corresponds to the term osteoid volume, which means the percentage of nonmineralized bone in relation to a unit volume of total bone tissue (Table 2). The volumetric density of the osteoid remains on the average, the same during life, except during the two first decades when higher values exist. MERZ and SCHENK (1970b) as well as COURPON (1972) reported similar results. Thus the surface extent of the osteoid seams increases with increasing age, the mean osteoid seam thickness decreases from 15 μ in the thirties to 12 μ in the eighties. MERZ and ŠCHENK (1970b) observed a decrease from 11 to 7 μ. JOHNSON et al. (1971) found in 100 μ thick ground sections a reduction of 6 μ (16 μ at middle age, 10 μ at higher age). The osteoid seam thickness of cancellous bone in the iliac crest was significantly greater

Table 1. Parameters of the volume and structure

Age	0–1	1–10	11–20	21–30
Number of cases	4	3	6	7
Volumetric density (V_v; %)	37.5 ± 3.8	23.0 ± 3.9	20.7 ± 3.1	20.4 ± 4.0
Specific surface (S/V; mm²/mm³)	20.2 ± 3.2	18.6 ± 6.2	20.9 ± 2.3	18.4 ± 3.2
Surface density (S_v; mm²/mm³)	7.356 ± 0.876	3.791 ± 0.232	4.081 ± 0.429	3.507 ± 0.272
Inactive surface (IS; %)	58.8 ± 5.7	65.7 ± 6.3	70.6 ± 2.3	76.2 ± 8.00
Surface density of inactive surface (S_{vis}; mm²/mm³)	4.350 ± 0.766	2.490 ± 0.258	2.887 ± 0.385	2.659 ± 0.514

Table 2. Parameters of the volume and structure

Age	0–1	1–10	11–20	21–30
Number of cases	4	3	6	7
Volumetric density of osteoid (V_{vo}; %)	2.4 ± 0.6	1.2 ± 0.3	1.1 ± 0.5	0.9 ± 0.2
Osteoid seam thickness ($\overline{S}$; μ)	11.3 ± 1.3	13.9 ± 5.0	13.3 ± 5.6	14.8 ± 3.6
Active seams (OS; %)	22.4 ± 8.1	6.8 ± 4.5	4.8 ± 2.2	4.5 ± 3.2
Inactive seams (IO; %)	10.9 ± 2.3	18.7 ± 3.8	17.6 ± 3.6	14.2 ± 3.0
Total extent of seams (OS; %)	30.8 ± 8.7	25.5 ± 8.0	20.4 ± 2.8	17.5 ± 7.2
Relative activity of osteoblasts (ROBA; %)	62.5 ± 16.1	24.4 ± 13.0	14.2 ± 11.7	14.8 ± 8.5
Surface density of seams (S_{vos}; mm²/mm³)	2.537 ± 0.989	0.867 ± 0.311	0.832 ± 0.152	0.602 ± 0.265

than in the rib. In any case an increased volumetric density of osteoid is indicative of a disturbance in the new bone formation. With a delayed mineralization or an increased synthesis of bone matrix, there occurs a desynchronization of these two mechanisms—an enlarged mass of nonmineralized bone is the result (MERZ and SCHENK, 1970b).

b) Osteoblasts and Osteoid Seams

The total extent of osteoid seams is about 10–25 % of the total bone surface (Fig. 11). The osteoid comprises the greatest extent in the first years of life. During the period of growth a remarkable bone remodeling can be observed. The minimal extent of osteoid seams (12.3 ± 5.8%) is seen between 40 and 50 years (Table 2). MERZ and SCHENK (1970b), however, observed this reduction one decade earlier. At higher age the surface extent of seams increases up to 24.7 ± 9.1% (MERZ and SCHENK, 1970b, 20.5 ± 14.3%; BORDIER and TUN CHOT, 1972, 19.0 ± 4.7%). BORDIER and TUN CHOT (1972) described a continous increase of the osteoid extent without the minimum in middle age. In contrast to the total extent of seams, the percentage of active seams of cancellous bone in relation to age. M ± SD

31–40	41–50	51–60	61–70	71–80	81–90
7	6	11	14	10	6
20.0 ± 3.2	19.9 ± 4.6	18.6 ± 5.2	15.2 ± 4.8	14.2 ± 5.5	11.1 ± 3.3
20.2 ± 3.4	21.4 ± 5.6	18.6 ± 3.8	21.6 ± 4.4	21.0 ± 5.4	17.5 ± 4.3
3.447 ± 0.463	3.883 ± 0.283	3.246 ± 0.737	2.838 ± 0.594	2.582 ± 0.692	1.791 ± 0.587
79.4 ± 5.3	79.7 ± 4.7	73.6 ± 21.9	68.9 ± 13.3	72.6 ± 15.1	75.6 ± 3.8
2.733 ± 0.411	3.097 ± 0.349	2.595 ± 0.551	1.915 ± 0.533	1.540 ± 0.416	1.344 ± 0.402

of new bone formation in relation to age. M ± SD

31–40	41–50	51–60	61–70	71–80	81–90
7	6	11	14	10	6
0.7 ± 0.3	0.8 ± 0.5	0.5 ± 0.3	0.7 ± 0.4	0.7 ± 0.6	0.7 ± 0.4
13.0 ± 4.2	15.2 ± 5.6	11.9 ± 3.7	12.1 ± 5.4	14.2 ± 6.9	13.4 ± 4.6
2.1 ± 0.6	1.6 ± 0.9	1.7 ± 1.3	1.9 ± 1.1	0.9 ± 0.6	2.4 ± 1.9
14.1 ± 4.9	10.7 ± 5.8	11.4 ± 4.8	22.7 ± 8.9	19.9 ± 9.7	18.5 ± 4.4
15.3 ± 4.8	12.3 ± 5.8	13.2 ± 4.6	24.7 ± 9.1	20.9 ± 9.9	20.9 ± 5.1
13.9 ± 4.3	12.3 ± 8.2	16.7 ± 9.3	9.1 ± 7.3	5.6 ± 4.4	14.1 ± 11.3
0.532 ± 0.192	0.473 ± 0.225	0.438 ± 0.213	0.595 ± 0.335	0.567 ± 0.256	0.349 ± 0.179

(osteoid with osteoblasts) decreases from 22.4 ± 8.1 % in the first decade to 0.9 ± 0.6 % in the eighth (Fig. 12). MERZ and SCHENK (1970b) also observed a decrease of active seams, but to a smaller degree. This difference may be explained by different environmental factors. For instance, the tap water of Basel contains an artificial addition of fluoride not found in the tap water in Hamburg or in the North of Germany. Fluoride stimulates osteoblastic activity (REUTTER et al., 1970) and an influence of the fluoride addition in Switzerland may cause the differences described over a long period. In addition, in Switzerland, for instance, there is a much higher consumption of foods rich in calcium such as milk and milk products, and the calcium intake influences the balance of the skeletal system (HARRISON et al., 1961; HAAS, 1966; NORDIN, 1964). In contrast to the decrease of active seams, the surface extent of inactive seams (osteoid without osteoblasts) increases with increasing age. This may be the result of a delay in the secondary mineralization (MERZ and SCHENK, 1970b; BORDIER and TUN CHOT, 1972). The increase begins in the 5th or 6th decade and could be the result of the development of atherosclerosis in all organs, especially in the kidney, due to a reduced blood supply and a reduction of the kidney parenchyma. Thus the kidney produces active metabolites

Table 3. Parameters of the structure of

Age	0–1	1–10	11–20	21–30
Number of cases	4	3	6	7
Howship's lacunae with osteoclasts (HO; %)	3.2 ± 1.1	2.5 ± 1.5	3.2 ± 2.1	2.5 ± 1.5
Howship's lacunae without osteoclasts (HE; %)	5.4 ± 1.6	5.7 ± 1.7	5.9 ± 2.0	3.6 ± 1.1
Total Howship's lacunae (HT; %)	9.3 ± 2.8	9.8 ± 1.5	$9.0 \pm 3,7$	6.1 ± 1.9
Relative osteoclastic activity (ROCA; %)	34.7 ± 2.1	25.0 ± 13.3	32.2 ± 11.9	$39.1 \pm 15,0$
Index of osteoclasts (OI)	14.3 ± 4.6	13.0 ± 9.9	13.8 ± 8.6	11.4 ± 5.7
Surface density of total Howship's lacunae (S_{vht}; mm²/mm³)	0.735 ± 0.098	0.369 ± 0.039	0.352 ± 0.058	0.208 ± 0.058

Table 4. Changes of the percentage of small and large
cancellous bone (iliac crest) in relation to age. In undecal-

Age	1–10	11–20	21–30
Number of cases	3	6	7
Small osteocytes (%)	54.7 ± 4.9	55.9 ± 14.0	46.7 ± 7.7
Large osteocytes (%)	39.8 ± 4.5	35.4 ± 15.2	42.2 ± 10.2
Empty lacunae (%)	8.2 ± 1.0	8.8 ± 5.5	11.1 ± 3.8

of vitamin D by hydrolyzation of 25–hydroxycholecalciferol to 1.25-dihydroxy-cholecalciferol (Deluca, 1971; Dambacher*et al.*, 1972a). This reaction is less in old age owing to the relative lack of kidney tissue. 1,25-dihydroxychole-calciferol is the active metabolite of vitamin D on bone tissue. When too little of this metabolite is produced, the result may be an increase of inactive seams due to a delay of the secondary mineralization. In vitamin D-deficiency, however, primary and secondary mineralization is incomplete whereas the matrix synthesis is normal. This results in broad osteoid seams with a surface extent of up to one hundred percent. Thus the bone changes described above may be secondary to the ageing processes of other organs. Gutteridge*et al.* (1968) and Bullamore *et al.* (1970) found reduced intestinal calcium absorption after the 60th year. They believe that all people older than 80 years have severe osteomalacia. Probably the diminished calcium absorption from the intestine or the relative calcium deficiency is another process which induces the increased extent of inactive seams in old age.

3. Changes in Bone Resorption

a) Lacunae of Howship

The parameters of bone resorption are summarized in Table 3. The percentage of Howship's lacunae with osteoclasts decreases up to the 5th decade bone resorption in relation to age. $M \pm SD$

31–40	41–50	51–60	61–70	71–80	81–90
7	6	11	14	10	6
1.6 ± 1.0	1.1 ± 0.8	1.9 ± 1.1	1.5 ± 1.3	2.1 ± 1.8	2.3 ± 0.9
3.8 ± 1.6	6.5 ± 1.0	4.5 ± 1.6	4.9 ± 1.5	5.7 ± 3.3	3.2 ± 1.6
5.4 ± 2.3	7.5 ± 1.6	6.4 ± 2.5	6.5 ± 2.2	7.8 ± 4.9	5.5 ± 2.3
27.8 ± 9.5	16.0 ± 9.4	29.5 ± 9.7	22.0 ± 13.1	25.3 ± 9.4	41.4 ± 8.6
6.4 ± 2.7	5.3 ± 4.1	9.4 ± 5.5	7.5 ± 5.2	9.3 ± 7.5	9.8 ± 4.9
0.182 ± 0.069	0.295 ± 0.087	0.203 ± 0.069	0.161 ± 0.051	0.207 ± 0.079	0.098 ± 0.059

osteocytes as well as of empty osteocytic lacunae of the
cified sections 70 osteocytes were counted per case. $M \pm SD$

31–40	41–50	51–60	61–70	71–80	81–90
7	6	11	14	10	6
51.8 ± 6.8	36.5 ± 1.2	29.1 ± 10.5	36.9 ± 11.2	32.1 ± 17.5	23.3 ± 5.0
37.1 ± 3.4	42.6 ± 11.1	51.7 ± 13.3	44.2 ± 9.1	48.2 ± 10.9	53.8 ± 5.1
11.1 ± 3.1	20.9 ± 10.3	19.4 ± 11.0	14.0 ± 8.1	18.8 ± 8.0	20.2 ± 7.3

and slightly increases in the following periods (Fig. 13). These values are
surprisingly higher than those described by SCHENK *et al.* (1969). The percentage of empty lacunae is at a minimum between 30 and 40 years. Later an
increase with remarkable deviation of the mean value occurs (Fig. 13). The
extent of total Howship's lacunae shows the some tendency (Fig. 14). It is

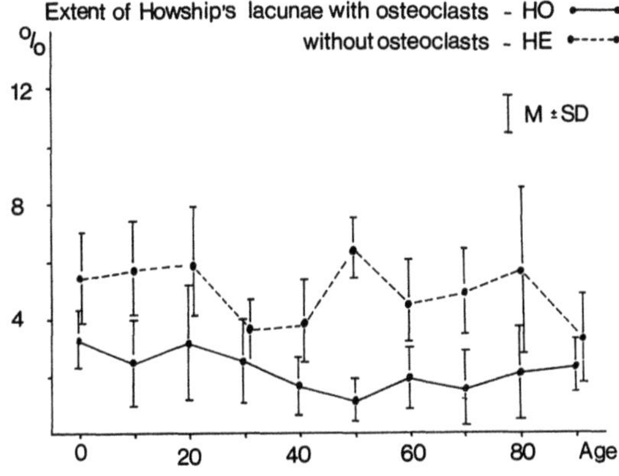

Fig. 13. Surface extent of Howship's lacunae with and without osteoclasts. There is a
slight increase of lacunae with osteoclasts at an advanced age. $M \pm SD$

interesting that the values of the total extent of Howship's lacunae are again similar to the published data of Schenk *et al.* (1969) in contrast to the relation of lacunae with osteoclasts described above. Bordier and Tun Chot (1972) found an increase of the resorption surface (total extent) up to more than 17 %. Such high percentage could never be observed in the own material. The total surface extent of lacunae, however, does not represent the actual resorption,

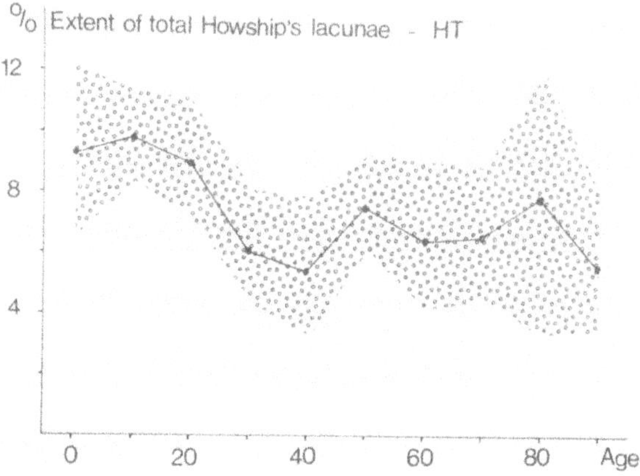

Fig. 14. Total surface of Howship's lacunae. The values remain almost unchanged in all decades. Shaded area indicates the standard deviation

because an increased number of empty lacunae is the result of a diminished new bone formation (Schenk *et al.*, 1969). In other words, the resorption places were not repaired by active osteoblasts. For investigation of actual bone resorption the number of osteoclasts is more important. Far more useful, however, would be the knowledge of the real activity of these cells. Unfortunately it has thus far been impossible to determine the resorption rate of the osteoclasts.

b) Activity of Osteoclasts

The number of osteoclasts in relation to the surface density, i.e. the index of osteoclasts, is at a minimum in the 5th decade and increases slightly in the following years. The surface density of total Howship's lacunae shows until the end of the growth period its highest value (0.352 ± 0.143 mm^2/mm^3). In the next two decades a decrease occurs. A second small rise takes place between ages 40 and 50 (Table 3). The general loss of bone mass begins after this period. Schenk *et al.* (1969) described a constant index of osteoclasts during all decades and suggested that the loss of bone mass was the consequence of the reduced formation of new bone only. Hioco (1966), Barer and Jowsey (1967) as well as Bordier and Tun Chot (1972) observed a gradual increase of bone resorption at an advanced age. Therefore they believed the development of osteoporosis to be the consequence of increased bone resorption. Our own observation led us to the supposition that after the 5th decade three processes of different degree cause the loss of bone mass. The slightly increased osteoclastic resorption reduces the cancellous bone. The considerable simultaneous decrease of osteoblastic activity (Fig. 15) enhances this bone rarefication by reduction of new bone formation. The delayed mineralization of the inactive seams may have an additional effect on the reduction of bone mass. Some osteoblasts compensate the bone reduction by a thickening of the main trabeculae of

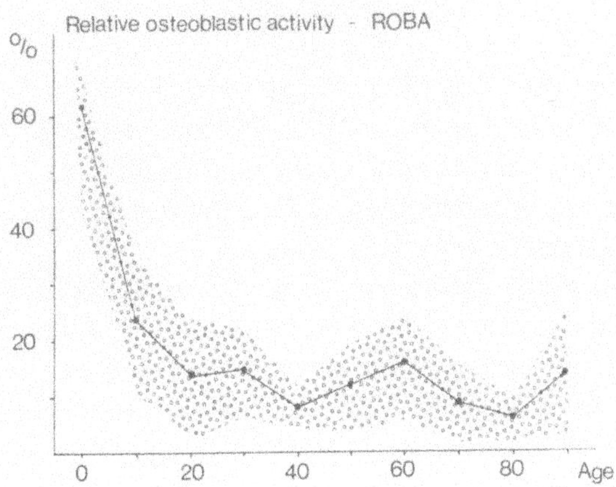

Fig. 15. Relative Osteoblastic activity in relation to age. Note the early decrease in the 2nd decade. The shaded area represents the standard deviation of the mean value.

cancellous bone (compensated hypertrophy) as described by EGER *et al.* (1965) as well as by SCHENK *et al.* (1969).

4. Changes in the Inactive Surface of Cancellous Bone

The percentage of inactive surface in relation to the total bone surface remains constant from the 10th to the 90th year. The absolute value (surface density of inactive surface) decreases, of course, from the 5th decade in correlation with the gradual loss of bone mass.

5. Changes in the Osteocytes

Besides the characteristic changes in the cancellous bone surfaces, the inner surfaces of bone show a special feature in relation to age. Thus, the size of the osteocytic lacunae changes as well as the number of the osteocytes per unit volume of mineralized bone. These changes were measured by estimating the percentage of small and large osteocytes as well as empty lacunae. After the 5th decade the percentage of large (bone resorbing?) osteocytes rises whereas a decrease of small (bone forming?) osteocytes takes place between the 4th and 6th decade. The empty osteocytic lacunae increase with advancing age (Table 4). FROST (1960a, 1960b) observed similar values in cortical bone of the long bones. BAUD and AUIL (1971) described a minimum of large osteo-

cytes between the 36th and 45th years, and a reduction of the small osteocytes after the 55th year measured in the lower jaw. Under pathological
conditions, for instance in primary and secondary hyperparathyroidism, the
number of large osteocytes increases (MEUNIER *et al.*, 1971). Probably in counting these cells a distinction may be drawn between normal and pathological
bone processes.

VI. Summary

The skeleton changes its structure and mass during human life due to
endogenous and exogenous factors. In addition, ageing processes of the extracellular substance and of the bone cells themselves play an important but in
detail unknown role. All of these factors result in a characteristic remodeling
of human cancellous bone in relation to age.

New methods, particularly bone biopsy procedures, histological preparation of undecalcified bone and the quantitative analysis for measuring the
volumes and surfaces of cancellous bone now allow a clearer insight into the
pathogenesis of bone diseases. Differentiation between physiological and
pathological changes can be made only when an exact knowledge of age-related
bone changes is available.

These age-related bone changes are characterized as follows:

1. The volumetric density of cancellous bone, i.e., the bone mass, shows
from the 4th to the 9th decade a gradual decrease of about 21% to 12%.

2. The surface density, the important surface for general metabolic processes between the bone and the marrow space, diminishes in the same degree.

3. As a consequence of so-called compensated hypertrophy, the specific
surface, i.e., the reciprocal value of the trabecula diameter, decreases slightly
at an advanced age. Osteoporosis develops if this process does not occur.

4. One of the most important pathogenic factors in reducing the bone mass
is an insuffiency of the osteoblasts at an advanced age.

5. The loss of bone substance might be enhanced due to a delay if mineralization resulting in an increase of the surface extent of inactive osteoid
seams (seams without osteoblasts).

6. The osteoclastic resorption shows a remarkable deviation of the mean
value during life. After the 5th decade there occurs a slight increase in the
extent of Howship's lacunae as well as in the index of osteoclasts. In agreement
with SCHENK *et al.* (1970a) it is supposed that this process plays a secondary
role in the development of bone rarefaction. Most important is the reduction
in formation of new bone.

7. The percentage of small and large osteocytes shows characteristic changes
at an advanced age. The number of large osteocytes increases, that of small
ones decreases.

When data concerning many parameters of bone remodeling, such as bone
structure, percentage of surfaces and bone cell activity, are available, a generalized osteopathy in border cases or in very early stages can be recognized.

In addition, a systematic study by the methods and parameters described above greatly facilitates the clarification of the pathogenesis of certain bone diseases.

References

ADAMS, P., DAVIES, G. T., SWEETNAM, P.: Osteoporosis and the effects of ageing on bone mass in elderly men and women. Quart. J. Med. **39**, 601 (1970).

ADAMS, P., DAVIES, G. T., SWEETNAM, P.: Cortical bone loss with age. Lancet **1971 II** 1201–1202.

ALTANESE, A. A., EDELSON, A. H., LORENZE, E., WEIN, E. H.: Quantitative radiographic survey technique for detection of bone loss. J. Amer. Geriat. Soc. **17**, 142 (1969).

AMTMANN, E., SCHMITT, H. P.: Über die Verteilung der Corticalisdichte im menschlichen Femurschaft und ihre Bedeutung für die Bestimmung der Knochenfestigkeit. Z. Anat. Entwickl.-Gesch. **127**, 25–41 (1968).

ARMAN, E., REIZENSTEIN, P.: Hand radioactivity after intraveneous injection of ⁴⁷C Effect of age and femoral neck fracture. Geriatrics **26**, 155–165 (1971).

ARNOLD, J. S., BARTLEY, M. H., TONT, S. A., JENKINS, D. P.: Skeletal changes in ageing and disease. Clin. Orthop. **49**, 17–38 (1966).

ATKINSON, P. J.: Variation in trabecular structure of vertebrae with age. Calcif. Tiss. Res. **1**, 24–32 (1967).

ATKINSON, P. J., WEATHERELL, J. A., WEIDMANN, S. M.: Changes in density of the human femoral cortex with age. J. Bone Jt. Surg. **844**, 498–502 (1962).

ATKINSON, P. J., WOODHEAD, C.: Changes in human mandibular structure with age. Arch. oral. Biol. **13**, 1453–1463 (1968).

BALL, J.: A simple method of defining osteoid in undecalcified sections. J. clin. Path. **10**, 281 (1957).

BARER, M., JOWSEY, J.: Bone formation and resorption in normal human rib. Clin. Orthop. **52**, 241–247 (1967).

BARTELHEIMER, H.: Die klinische Bedeutung der Knochenbiopsie. Verh. dtsch. Ges. Path. **47**, 145 (1963).

BARTELHEIMER, H., SCHMITT-ROHDE, J. M.: Die Biopsie des Knochens als differential-diagnostische klinische Methode. Klin. Wschr. **35**, 429 (1957).

BARZEL, U. S.: The effect of excessive acid feeding on bone. Calcif. Tiss. Res. **4**, 94–100 (1969).

BAUD, C. A.: Morphologie et structure inframicroscopique des osteocytes. Acta anat. (Basel) **51**, 209–225 (1962).

BAUD, C. A.: Structure et fonctions des osteocytes dans les conditions normales et sous l'influence de l'extrait parathyroiden. Schweiz. med. Wschr. **98**, 717–720 (1968).

BAUD, C. A., AUIL, E.: Osteocyte differential count in normal human alveolar bone. Acta anat. (Basel) **78**, 321–327 (1971).

BAUER, G. C. H., CARLSSON, A., LINDQUIST, B.: Use of isotopes in clinical studies of skeletal metabolism. Radioaktive Isotope Klin. Forsch. **3**, 25 (1958).

BECK, J. S., NORDIN, J.: Histological assessment of osteoporosis by iliac crest biopsy. J. Path. Bact. **80**, 391 (1960).

BÉLANGER, L. F.: Osteocytic osteolysis. Calcif. Tiss. Res. **4**, 1–12 (1969).

BELL, G. H., DUNBAR, O., BECK, J. S.: Variations in strength of vertebrae with age and their relation to osteoporosis. Calcif. Tiss. Res. **1**, 75–86 (1967).

BINSWANGER, U., FISCHER, J., SCHENK, R., MERZ, W.: Osteopathie bei chronischer Niereninsuffizienz. Dtsch. med. Wschr. **49**, 1914 (1971).

BÖRNER, W., GREHN, S., MOLL, E., RAUH, E., SEYBOLD, K.: Altersphysiologische und pathologische Veränderungen der Dichte und Dicke des Fingerknochens. Radiologische Messung mit einem ¹²⁵J-Profilscanner an 223 Frauen. Fortschr. Röntgenstr. **116**, 552–558 (1972).

BOLLET, A. J.: Osteoporosis, or the osteoporosities? Amer. J. med. Sci. **256**, 271–278 (1968).

BORDIER, Ph. I., TUN CHOT, S.: Quantitative histology of metabolic bone disease. Clin. Endocrin. Metab. **1**, 197–215 (1972).

Boukhris, R., Becker, K. L.: Calcification of the aorta and osteoporosis. J. Amer. med. Ass. **219**, 1307–1311 (1972).

Bullamore, J. R., Gallagher, J. L., Wilkinson, R., Nordin, B. E. C.: Effect of age on calcium absorption. Lancet **1970 II**, 535–537.

Burkhardt, R.: Präparative Voraussetzungen zur klinischen Histologie des menschlichen Knochenmarkes. Blut **14**, 30–45 (1966).

Burr, I. M., Sizonenko, P. C., Kapla, S. L., Grumbach, M. M.: Hormonal changes in puberty: I. Correlation of serum luteinizing hormone and follicle stimulating hormone with stages of puberty, testicular size, and bone age in normal boys. Pediat. Res. **4**, 25–35 (1970).

Chalmers, J., Weaver, J. K.: Cancellous bone: Its strength and changes with aging and an evaluation of some methods for measuring its mineral content. J. Bone Surg. A **48**, 299–308 (1966).

Courpron, P.: Donées histologiques quantitatives sur le viellissement osseux humain. Thèse (unpublished), Lyon 1972.

Currey, J. D.: The mechanical consequences of variation in the mineral content of bone. J. Biomech. **2**, 1–11 (1969).

Dambacher, M. A., Girard, J., Haas, H. G.: Die Vitamin D "Hormone". Neue Erkenntnisse über Stoffwechsel und Therapie. Internist (Berl.) **13**, 125 (1972a).

Dambacher, M. A., Scriba, P. C., Haas, H. G.: Epithelkörperchen und metabolische Osteopathien. Teil I B der Endokrinologie der Praxis, Hrsg. K. Schwarz und P. C. Scriba. München: Lehmann 1972b.

Dambacher, M. A., Steiger, U., Haas, H. G.: Osteoporose — neue Aspekte der Pathophysiologie und der Therapie. Med. Klin. **66**, 33–39 (1971).

Delesse, M. A.: Procédé mécanique pour déterminer la composition des roches. 3e éd. Paris: F. Sary 1866,

Delling, G.: Über eine vereinfachte Methylmethacrylat-Einbettung für unentkalkte Knochenschnitte. Beitr. path. Anat. **145**, 100–105 (1972).

Delling, G.: Quantitative Auswertung von Skeletveränderungen bei chronischer Hämodialyse. Verh. dtsch. Ges. Path. **56**, 436–438 (1972).

Delling, G.: Altersabhängige histologische Veränderungen der Beckenkammspongiosa. Kli. Wschr. (in press) 1973.

Delling, G., Donath, K.: Morphometrische, elektronenmikroskopische und physikalisch-chemische Untersuchungen über die experimentelle Osteoporose bei chronischer Azidose. Virchows Arch. Abt. A **358**, 321–330 (1973).

Deluca, H. F.: Vitamin D: A new look at an old vitamin. Nutr. Rev. **29**, 179–181 (1971).

Dequeker, J.: Bone loss in normal and pathological conditions. Leuven: Leuven Univ. Press 1972.

Dequeker, J., Remans, J., Franssen, R., Waes, J.: Ageing pattern of trabecular and cortical bone and their relationship. Calcif. Tiss. Res. **7**, 23–30 (1971).

Donath, K., Delling, G.: Elektronenmikroskopische Darstellung der periosteocytären Matrix durch Ultradünnschnitt-EDTA-Entkalkung. Virchows Arch. Abt. A **354**, 305–311 (1971).

Doyle, F., Brown, J., Lachance, C.: Relation between bone mass and muscle weight. Lancet **1970 I**, 391–393.

Dunnill, M. S., Anderson, J. A., Whitehead, R.: Quantitative histological studies on age changes in bone. J. Path. Bact. **94**, 275–291 (1967).

Eger, W.: Pathologische Anatomie der Osteoporose unter besonderer Berücksichtigung der Mineralstoffwechselvorgänge im Knochengewebe. Verh. dtsch. Ges. inn. Med. **71**, 533–568 (1965).

Eger, W., Gerner, H. J., Kämmerer, H.: Bau und Dichte der menschlichen Spongiosa in Rippe und Becken als Ausdruck der statischen Funktion. Arch. orthop. Unfall-Chir. **62**, 97–112 (1967).

Eger, W., Götz, F., Kämmerer, H.: Herstellung von Dünnschliffen aus Knochen und Weichgewebe nach Markierung mit Tetracyclinen. Langenbecks Arch. klin. Chir. **306**, 205–214 (1964).

Ellis, H. A., Peart, K. H.: Quantitative observations on mineralized and nonmineralized bone in the iliac crest. J. clin. Path. **25**, 277 (1972).

Exton-Smith, A. N., Payne, P. R., Wheeler, E. F.: Cortical bone-loss with age. Lancet **1971 II**, 1377.

FRANKS, L. M.: Theories of ageing: cellular aspects. Proc. roy. Soc. Med. **65**, 372–373 (1972).

FROST, H. M.: In vivo osteocyte death. J. Bone Jt Surg. A **42**, 138–143 (1960a).

FROST, H. M.: Micropetrosis. J. Bone Jt Surg. A **42**, 144–150 (1960b).

FROST, H. M.: Bone remodelling dynamics. Springfield, Illinois: Thomas 1963.

FROST, H. M.: The bone dynamics in osteoporosis and osteomalacia. Springfield, Illinois: Thomas 1966.

FROST, H. M.: Tetracycline bone labelling in anatomy. Amer. J. Anthrop. **29**, 183–196 (1968).

FROST, H. M.: Tetracycline-based histological analysis of bone remodelling. Calcif. Tiss. Res. **3**, 211–237 (1969).

GARN, M. S., ROHMANN, C. G., WAGNER, B.: Bone loss as a general phenomenon in man. Fed. Proc. **26**, 1729–1736 (1967).

GARNER, A., BALL, J.: Quantitative observations on mineralized and unmineralized bone in chronic renal azotemia and intestinal malabsorption syndrome. J. Path. Bact. **91**, 554 (1966).

GLIMCHER, M.: A basic architectural principle in the organization of mineralized tissue. Clin. Orthop. **61**, 16–36 (1968).

GOLDNER, J.: A modification of the Masson trichromtechnique for routine laboratory purpose. Amer. J. Path. **14**, 237–243 (1938).

GREEN, G. H.: A simple method for histological examination of bone marrow particles using hydroxyethyl methacrylate embedding. J. clin. Path. **23**, 640–643 (1970).

GRYFE, C. J., EXTON-SMITH, A. N., PAYNE, P. R., WHEELER, E. F.: Pattern of development of bone in childhood and adolescence. Lancet **1971 I**, 523–526.

GUDMUNDSSON, H., WOODHOUSE, N. J. Y.: Regulation of plasma calcium in man: the influence of parathyroid hormone and calcitonin. Hormones **2**, 26–39 (1971).

GUTTERTRIDGE, D. H., ROBINSON, C. J., JOPLIN, G. F.: Delayed strontium absorption in postmenopausal osteoporosis and osteomalacia. Clin. Sci. **34**, 351–363 (1968).

HAAS, H. G.: Knochenstoffwechsel- und Parathyreoidea-Erkrankungen. Stuttgart: Thieme 1966.

HALL, B. K.: Histogenesis and morphogenesis of bone. Clin. Orthop. **74**, 249–268 (1971).

HALL, D. A.: Theories of ageing: extracellular aspects. Proc. roy. Soc. Med. **65**, 671–672 (1972).

HARRISON, M., FRASER, R., MULLAN, B.: Calcium metabolism in osteoporosis. Acute and long-term responses to increased calcium intake. Lancet **1961 I**, 1015–1019.

HENNIG, A.: Bestimmung der Oberfläche beliebig geformter Körper mit besonderer Anwendung auf Körperhaufen im mikroskopischen Bereich. Mikroskopie **11**, 1–20 (1956).

HENNIG, A.: Kritische Betrachtungen zur Volumen- und Oberflächenmessung in der Mikroskopie. Zeiss Werkzeitschr. **30**, 78–86 (1958).

HERRING, G. M.: The chemical structure of tendon, cartilage, dentin and bone matrix. Clin. Orthop. **60**, 261–299 (1968).

HEUCK, F.: Allgemeine Morphologie und Biodynamik des Knochens im Röntgenbild. Fortschr. Röntgenstr. **112**, 354–365 (1970).

HIOCO, D.: Physiopathologie und Therapie der Osteoporose. Dtsch. med. Wschr. **91**, 1079 (1966).

HIRSCH, TH. v., BOELLARD, J. W.: Methacrylsäureester als Einbettungsmittel in der Histologie. Z. wiss. Mikr. **64**, 24–29 (1958).

HRUZA, Z., WACHTLOVA, M.: Diminution of bone blood flow and capillary network in rats during aging. J. Geront. **24**, 315–320 (1969).

JANDE, S. S.: Fine structural study of osteocytes and their surrounding bone matrix with respect to their age in young chicks. J. Ultrastruct. Res. **37**, 279–300 (1971).

JOHNSON, K. A., RIGGS, B. L., KELLY, P. J., JOWSEY, J.: Osteoid tissue in normal and osteoporotic individuals. Clin. Endocr. Metab. **33**, 745–751 (1971).

JOWSEY, J.: Age changes in human bone. Clin. Orthop. **17**, 210–218 (1960).

JOWSEY, J., KELLY, P. J., RIGGS, B. L., BIANCO, A. L., SCHOLZ, D. A., GERSHON-COHEN, J.: Quantitative microradiographic studies of normal and osteoporotic bone. J. Bone Jt Surg. A **47**, 785–806 (1965).

KIENITZ, M.: Tetracycline in Knochen und Zähnen. Dtsch. med. Wschr. **90**, 1298 (1965).

KNEESE, K. H.: Knochenstruktur als Verbundbau. Stuttgart: Thieme 1958.

Kneese, K. H.: Zell- und Faserstruktur des Knochengewebes. Acta anat. (Basel) **53**, 369–394 (1963).

Korenchevsky, V.: Physiological and pathological ageing, ed.: Bourne, G. H., Basel: S. Karger 1961.

Krokowski, E.: Möglichkeiten zur Bestimmung des Skelett-Calciumgehaltes in der Klinik. Dtsch. med. Wschr. **91**, 60 (1966).

Kuhlenkordt, F.: Osteoporose. Verh. dtsch. Ges. Orthop. **57**, 221 (1970).

Kuhlenkordt, F., Wieners, H., Gocke, H.: Skelettuntersuchungen bei Diabetikern bis zum 45. Lebensjahr. Dtsch. med. Wschr. **91**, 1913 (1966).

Lozano-Tonkin, C.: Die Knochenbiopsie und ihre Indikation in der Inneren Medizin. Münch. med. Wschr. **110**, 2213–2219 (1968).

Magill, H., Gunning, B.: A simple microtome capable of cutting sections of plastic-embedded material down to 1 μm in thickness. J. Microscopy **89**, 217–223 (1968).

Merz, W. A.: Die Streckenmessung an gerichteten Strukturen im Mikroskop und ihre Anwendung zur Bestimmung von Oberflächen-Volumen-Relationen im Knochengewebe. Mikroskopie **22**, 132–142 (1967).

Merz, W. A., Schenk, R. K.: Quantitative structural analysis of human cancellous bone. Acta anat. (Basel) **74**, 140–149 (1970a).

Merz, W. A., Schenk, R. K.: A quantitative histological study on bone formation in human cancellous bone. Acta anat. (Basel) **76**, 1–15 (1970b).

Meunier, P., Bernard, J., Vignon, G.: The measurement of periosteocytic enlargement in primary and secondary hyperparathyroidism. Israel J. med. Sci. **7**, 482–485 (1971).

Motta, C.: Zum Problem des Knochenwachstums beim Fehlen eines physiologischen Widerlagers. Z. Orthop. **104**, 506–512 (1968).

Müller, J., Schenk, R. K.: Knochenstruktur und Knochenumbau. Melsunger med. Mitt. **40**, 45–68 (1966).

Mueller, K. H., Trias, A., Ray R. D.: Bone density and composition. J. Bone Surg. A **48**, 140–148 (1966).

Muenzenberg, K. J., Gebhardt, M.: Tetracyclin und Knochenkollagen. Arch. orthop. Unfall-Chir. **67**, 211–216 (1970).

Newton, H. F., Morgan, D. B.: Osteoporosis: Disease or senescence. Lancet **1968 I**, 232–233.

Nilsson, B. O.: Parity and osteoporosis. Surg. Gynec. Obstet. **129**, 27–28 (1969).

Nordin, B. E. C.: The pathogenesis of osteoporosis. Lancet **1961 I**, 1011–1014.

Nordin, B. E. C.: The application of basic science to osteoporosis. In: Bone biodynamics, ed. H. M. Frost, p. 521–542, Boston: Littl. Brown 1964.

Nordin, B. E. C.: Hormones and calcium metabolism. In: Calcif. Tiss. 1965, Proc. 3rd European Symposium on Calcif. Tiss. eds H. Fleisch, H. J. J. Blackwood, M. Owen, Berlin—Heidelberg—New York: Springer 1966.

Nordin, B. E. C., MacGregor, J., Smith, D. A.: The incidence of osteoporosis in normal women: its relation to age and the menopause. Quart. J. Med. **35**, 25–38 (1966).

Olah, A. J., Schenk, R. K.: Veränderungen des Knochenvolumens und des Knochenanbaues in menschlichen Rippen und ihre Abhängigkeit zum Alter und Geschlecht. Acta anat. (Basel) **72**, 584–602 (1969).

Pauwels, F.: Über die Verteilung der Spongiosadichte im coxalen Femurende und ihre Bedeutung für die Lehre zum funktionellen Bau des Knochens, Morph. Jb. **95**, 35–54 (1954).

Pauwels, F.: Gesammelte Abhandlungen zur Funktionellen Anatomie des Bewegungsapparates. Berlin—Heidelberg—New York: Springer. 1965.

Pommer, G.: Untersuchungen über Osteomalazie und Rachitis nebst Beiträgen zur Kenntnis der durchbohrenden Gefäße. Leipzig: Vogel 1885.

Pommer, G.: Über Osteoporose, ihren Ursprung und ihre differentialdiagnostische Bedeutung. Langenbecks Arch. klin. Chir. **136**, 1 (1925).

Popowitz, M., Johnston, A. D.: Osteoporosis: Controlled methods of measurement. Clin. Orthop. **74**, 185–195 (1971).

Reutter, F. W., Siebermann, R., Pajarola, M.: Fluoride in osteoporosis. In: Vischer Th. L. (ed.) Fluoride in medicine. Bern: H. Huber 1970.

Robinson, R. A., Elliott, S. R.: The water content of bone. J. Bone Jt Surg. A **39**, 167–187 (1957).

ROCKOFF, S. D., KAYE, H., ARMSTRONG, J. D., STANSEL, H. C.: Effect of increased bone blood flow on bone metabolism. Invest. Radiol. 4, 230–235 (1969).

SACKER, L. S., NORDIN, B. E. C.: A simple bone biopsy needle. Lancet 1954 I, 347.

SAVILLE, P. D.: Changes in bone mass with age and alcoholism. J. Bone Jt Surg. A 47, 492–499 (1965).

SAVILLE, P. D., WHYTE, B. S.: Muscle and bone hypertrophy. Positive effect of running exercise in the rat. Clin. Orthop. 65, 81–88 (1969).

SCHENK, R. K.: Zur histologischen Verarbeitung von unentkalktem Knochen. Acta anat. (Basel) 60, 3–19 (1965).

SCHENK, R. K., MERZ, W. A.: Histologisch-morphometrische Untersuchungen über Altersatrophie und senile Osteoporose in der Spongiosa des Beckenkammes. Dtsch. med. Wschr. 94, 206 (1969).

SCHENK, R. K., MERZ, W. A., MÜLLER, J.: A quantitative histological study on bone resorption in human cancellous bone. Acta anat. (Basel) 74, 44–53 (1969).

SCHERFT, J. P.: The lamina limitans of the organic matrix of calcified cartilage and bone. J. Ultrastruct. Res. 38, 318–331 (1972).

SCHUBERT, M., PRAS, M.: Ground substance proteinpolysaccharides and the precipitation of calcium phosphate. Clin. Orthop. 60, 235–255 (1968).

SHIMO, R.: Method of preparing thin undecalcified serial sections of calcified tissue and technological observations. Jikeikai med. J. 15, 202–216 (1968).

SISSONS, H. A.: Histological studies of normal and osteoporotic bone. In: L'osteoporose, ed. HIOCO, D., p. 3–6. Paris: Masson 1964.

SIZONENKO, P. C., BURR, I. M., KAPLAN, S. L., GRUMBACH, M. M.: Hormonal changes in puberty. II. Pediat. Res. 4, 36–45 (1970).

SKOSEY, J. L.: Some basic aspects of bone metabolism in relation to osteoporosis. Med. Clin. N. Amer. 54, 141–152 (1970).

TALMAGE, R. V.: Morphological and physiological considerations in a new concept of calcium transport in bone. Amer. J. Anat. 129, 467–476 (1970).

TROTTER, M. BROMAN, G. E., PETERSON, R. R.: Densities of bones of white and negro skeletons. J. Bone Jt Surg. A 42, 50 (1960).

URIST, M. R., GURVEY, M. S., FAREED, O. D.: Long-term observations on aged women with pathological osteoporosis. In: Osteoporosis, ed. U. S. BARZEL. New York: Grune & Stratton 1970.

URIST, M. R., McLEAN, F. C.: Recent advances in physiology of bone. Part II. The parathyroid glands and bone. J. Bone Jt Surg. A 45, 1314–1320 (1963).

VITALLI, H. P.: Knochenerkrankungen, Histologie und Klinik. Basel: Sandoz 1970.

VOST, A.: Osteoporosis. A necropsy study of vertebrae and iliac crest. Amer. J. Path. 43, 143 (1963).

WAGNER, H.: Präsenile Osteoporose. Stuttgart: Thieme 1965.

WAKAMATSY, E., SISSONS, H. A.: The cancellous bone of the iliac crest. Calcif. Tiss. Res. 4, 147–161 (1969).

WEBER, D. A., GREENBERG, E. J., DIMICH, A., KENNY, P. J., ROTHSCHILD, E. O., MYERS, W. P. L., LAUGHLIN, J. S.: Kinetics of radionuclides used for bone studies. J. nucl. Med. 10, 8–17 (1969).

WEST, R. R., REED, G. W.: The measure of bone mineral in vivo by photon beam scanning. Brit. J. Radiol. 43, 886–893 (1970).

WILLIAMS, J. A., NICHOLSON, G. T.: A modified bone biopsy drill for outpatient use. Lancet 1963 II, 1408.

WILLS, M. R.: Fundamental physiological role of parathyroid hormone in acid-base homeostasis. Lancet 1970 II, 802–804.

WOODS, C. G., MORGAN, D. B., PATERSON, C. R., GOSSMANN, H. H.: Measurement of osteoid in bone biopsy. J. Path. Bact. 95, 441 (1968).

WU, K., SCHUBECK, K. E., FROST, H. M., VILANUEVA, A.: Haversian bone formation rates determined by a new method in a mastodon, and in human diabetes mellitus and osteoporosis. Calcif. Tiss. Res. 6, 204–219 (1970).

ZAMBERLAND, J., BLOCK, M., VATTER, A., TRENNER, L.: An adaption methacrylate embedding for routine histopathological use. Blood 33, 444–451 (1969).

Department of Pathology, University of Zürich, Switzerland, and
Department of Pathology, University of Düsseldorf, West-Germany

Perinatal and Newborn Deaths

Necropsy Findings in 970 Term, Preterm, and Small-for-Date Births

GISELA MOLZ*

With 3 Figures

Contents

The *newborn period* begins with the first day of life and lasts until the end
of the fourth week. The period between the 28th week of pregnancy and the
completed 7th day of life is defined as the *perinatal period*. Neonatal mor-

* Department of Anatomy, University of Zürich, Switzerland

tality is concerned only with live births, whereas *perinatal mortality* also includes infants dying before or during birth.

There is a high mortality rate exhibited during the perinatal and newborn periods: in 1958, the perinatal mortality rate in England and Wales was 35 per thousand. An investigation in the German Federal Republic in 1951 showed that of infants which die within their first year of life, 71 % die during the first month and 35 % on the first day.

For many years attempts have been made to ascertain the etiology of perinatal and neonatal mortality. The most comprehensive investigations were performed in Great Britain: of 7117 stillbirths or infants dying within the first month of life in March, April and May 1958, 5295 were available for necropsy, and the pathological findings were analyzed.

Stimulated by this excellent and thorough survey, we prepared the following analysis of the proportion of term, preterm and small-for-date births in terms of perinatal and neonatal mortality on the basis of 970 necropsies.

A. Materials and Methods

Autopsies were performed by the same pathologist on 130 stillbirths and 840 newborns who died between the 1st and 28th day. A standard "en bloc" technique was used for removal of thoracic and abdominal viscera. The examinations were complete, except in the case of a three-week-old newborn with sacral teratoma where the head section was refused.

The Institute of Pathology, Düsseldorf University supplied 289 necropsies (October 1957—March 1961), the cases coming from Lying-In and Children's Hospital and from other hospitals in the town and the surrounding areas. The other 681 necropsies (December 1963—August 1970) came from the Institute of Pathology, Zürich University, from the University Lying-In and Children's Hospital as well as from municipal and local area hospitals.

The histological analysis, particularly of the Zürich cases, is based on extensive examination of all organs: all paired organs, all endocrine organs, the parotid gland and bones were examined. *Perinatal* and *neonatal deaths* are divided according to single or multiple births and are analyzed under three headings:

I) State of maturity, sex, order of birth, mortality of first-born child and complications of labor.

II) Differentiation between stillbirth and newborn deaths, determination among the liveborns of the death rate on the first day, during the first three days, at the end of the first week and in the late neonatal period.

III) Selection of the primary necropsy findings, comparison of the primary necropsy findings in case of term, preterm and small-for-date births and a of the fundamental causes of death of the perinatal and neonatal periods.

B. Subdivision A: Singletons

I. Maturity, Sex, Order of Birth, Mortality of First-Born Child, Complications of Labor

1. Maturity

Duration of gestation is decisive. The term gestation is defined as the duration of amenorrhea in complete weeks, calculated from the first day of the last menstrual period.

In cases in which the dates were uncertain, length of gestation was determined by measurement and development of the child and by histologic examination of the organs.

Preterm births occur before expiration of a full 37-week gestation period;
Immature births, before 28 weeks of gestation;
Term births occur between the 38th and 41th weeks of gestation, and
Postmature births, after a pregnancy of 42 weeks or more.

Small-for-date includes term or preterm births whose development is retarded in comparison to the length of gestation. The underdevelopment is expressed not only in low birth weight and short stature but also in delayed morphologic development of the internal organs.

Results. Of 874 singletons, *term births* (338) and *preterm births* (332) were numerically almost equal, each group representing approximately 38%.

Small-for-date births (204) comprised 28%. Within this group the distribution by weeks of gestation was almost equal to that in the group of term (104) or preterm (100) births. The proportion of *immature* (75) to preterm births was 1:4. The 18 *postmature births* constituted such a small group that they were not considered separately; 15 were included in the term births and 3 in the small-for-date births.

The percentage of preterm births was distinctly lower than in other reported series: NEUWEILER and LUTZIGER (1966) indicated 69.2% preterm births, DHOM and KAFFARNIK (1958), 58%, NESBITT and ANDERSON (1956), 54%. These investigators did not, however, differentiate between single and multiple births or between preterm and small-for-date births. Because of a maximum of 80% preterm births among the twins, we separated single and multiple births. The warning given by PFAUNDLER (1941) that "it is entirely incorrect to consider a newborn as 'preterm' if and because its birth weight is less than 2500 grams" proves itself true in the latest metabolic examination of newborn infants. Thus for instance DAVIS *et al.* (1969) showed that small-for-date births have fewer reserves of glycogen, protein and fat than "true" preterm infants of equal weights. NESBITT and ANDERSON (1956) did not include immature infants (under 1000 grams). We have included these because every fourth preterm birth was by our definition immature.

2. Sex

Of the 874 singleton stillbirths and newborn deaths, 505 were male and 369 female, i.e., 57.7%:49.2%.

The percentage of boys rose to 60% among the preterm (199:133) and term (202:135) births. The preponderance of males reached a maximum at birth weights of over 4000 grams, 22 of the 25 babies being males. The sex ratio was equal in small-for-date births (104:100). These results are in accordance with the results of BUTLER and BONHAM (1963) who reported 55.3% male infants and 44.7% female infants. The preponderance of males amongst mature pregnancies was also reported by these authors. KOLB (1964) found the same relation in preterm births.

3. Order of Birth—Mortality of the First-Born Child

At the beginning of this century WESTERGAARD (s. PFAUNDLER, 1941), a medical statistician, observed that "first-born infants are far more frequently stillborn, and, if liveborn, are also more frequently subject to early death than subsequently born infants". BUTLER and BONHAM (1963) observed a high proportion of first-born infants among stillbirths in the investigation they performed in England in 1958. Re-examination of the present survey of 90 stillbirths and 598 newborn deaths confirms WESTERGAARD's observation; the proportion of first-born infants is high (45–48%), while the figure for second-born infants is only approximately half as high. This phenomenon holds true for all groups.

Table 1. Order of birth within the individual maturity groups

Order of birth	Term		Preterm		Small-for-date	
	No.	%	No.	%	No.	%
1	116	45	123	47	86	48
2	72	28	77	29	48	27
3	40	15	30	11	25	15
4	19	7	15	5	9	5
5	5		11		1	
6	4		2		1	
7	—		—		1	
8	1		2		—	
	257		260		171	

4. Complications of Labor

The following analyses include abnormal presentations (110 infants) and assisted deliveries (113 infants). For each group, the percentage represents approximately 12% of the total for each group.

a) Abnormal Presentation

Breech presentations (96) predominated; transverse (5) or face (7) and brow (2) presentations were rare. Individual maturity groups were present to a variable degree: 31 term births (9.1%), 58 preterm births (17%) and 21 small-for-date births (10%).

BUTLER and BONHAM (1963) stated two important facts: (1), that premature breech delivery of an infant which weighs 2500 grams or less results in mortality rate which is five times higher than that when the baby weighs more than 2500 grams; (2), that in all vaginal breech deliveries, the mortality rate of children of multiparous mothers is higher than that of the primipara. In our study, of the 96 breech deliveries, 34 are first-born, 54 later-born infants, and in 8 cases the order of birth was unknown.

Obstetrical intervention such as Caesarean section, forceps and vacuum delivery or manual extraction was necessary in every fourth case, and in term births, in every second case. The usual manual aids including Brachts delivery were not listed among obstetrical operations by BRETSCHER (1967). In the present survey, 2 newborn deaths were due to manual aids, so that these are also taken into account.

Detailed analysis of obstetrical intervention in term, preterm and small-for-date births is given in Table 2.

Table 2. Obstetrical intervention in abnormal presentation in term, preterm and small-for-date births

Maturity	Extract.	Caesarean sect.	Forceps	Vacuum	Manual aid
Term	4	8	1	4	4
Preterm	7	3			9
Small-for-date	2	2			4

b) Assisted Deliveries

Among the babies with vertex presentation, there were 113 with assisted deliveries. Caesarean sections (84) were predominant; forceps (14) and vacuum delivery (15) were of equal frequency. The incidence of term births (54) accounted for 16 %, of preterm births (37) and small-for-date births (22) for 10 %. A detailed analysis of fetal maternal involvement indicated that maternal reasons such as placenta praevia occurred with greater frequency in the preterm births (28 out of 37) whereas fetal involvement was as frequent as maternal in the term and small-for-date births.

II. Stillbirths and Newborn Deaths between the 1st to 28th days—Death Rate of Term, Preterm and Small-for-Date Births

1. Stillbirths

There were 712 singletons in the perinatal period of which 123 (16 %) were stillbirths.

This result represents a considerably lower percentage of stillbirths than that reported in the surveys of BUTLER and BONHAM (1963), 60 %, DHOM and KAFFARNIK (1958), 41.4 %, ZSCHOCH and MAHNKE (1968), 38.5 % and NEUWEILER and LUTZIGER (1966), 30 %. This discrepancy may be partially explained by the fact that selection took place in the Zürich cases, insofar as the cases observed in the Children's Hospital included *no* stillbirths. In a series of investigations (1956–63) at the Lying-In Hospital of Zürich University, MORF (1966) found 52 % stillbirths among 1061 perinatal deaths (multiple births included). In the Zürich Pathological Institute, a total of 1368 perinatal deaths were necropsied in the years 1964–70. The stillbirths—483—amounted to 35 %. However, in the individual years this percentage varied from 29–41 %.

Results. Of the 123 stillbirths, 65 were male and 58 female — 53 % : 47 %. There were 55 *term births*, 32 *preterm births* and 36 *small-for-date births*. Among the *postmature births* (6) 5 were born in the 43th week and one in the 45th week of gestation. *First-born children* constituted 60 %.

Nearly half of the stillbirths presented fresh at birth (57) and 66 were macerated. The times of death among fresh and macerated stillbirths are given in Table 3.

Table 3. Time of death for macerated and fresh stillbirths

Time of death	Stillbirths		Total
	macerated	fresh	
Antepartum	53	10	63
Intrapartum 1st stage	13	19	32
Intrapartum 2nd stage		28	28

As seen in Table 3, 50% died antepartum, 26% in the first stage and 23% in the second stage of labor. *Major lesions* are summarized in Table 4.

Table 4. Major lesions in fresh and macerated stillbirths

Major lesion	Fresh	Macerated
Malformations	7	4
Isoimmunization	4	15
Asphyxia with aspiration of meconium	18	13
Asphyxia with petechial hemorrhage	12	6
Asphyxia with subdural hemorrhage	7	3
Asphyxia with intraventricular hemorrhage	4	
Metabolic disease		3
Infection	1	1
Birth injuries	2	
No major lesion	1	21
Remainder	1	
Total cases	57	66

The following *malformations* were found: anencephalia (5), meningomyelocele with hydrocephalus (1), microcephalus (1), renal agenesis (1), esophageal atresia (1), left-side diaphragmatic agenesis (1) and a severe lesion of the heart (1).

Isoimmunization. Deaths resulted from blood group incompatibility (1) and severe hemolysis with afibrinogenemia in the mother (2). Intrauterine blood transfusion was performed in 4 children; in two of these cases the liver became necrotic after injuries caused by an instrument, in a third child the placental vein was injured. In the 4th child the testicles showed hemorrhagic infarction and pressure atrophy.

Asphyxia. Deaths in this category showed evidence of ante- or intrapartum asphyxia, namely excessive inhalation of amniotic fluid and/or meconium (31), widespread petechial hemorrhage on the visceral membranes (18), subdural hemorrhage (10) and intraventricular hemorrhage (4).

The *metabolic diseases* included fetopathia diabetica (2) and one adrenogenital syndrome (weight of suprarenal glands, 23 gm). The previously born brother (1st child) also died of an adrenogenital syndrome.

The *infections* were cases of staphylococcal sepsis and diffuse granulomatosis (without any recognizable cause).

Traumatic damage followed by death resulted after puncture of a placental vein during amnioscopy. Spinal and cranial fractures were sustained by one child during manual extraction in breech presentation.

In the category *no major lesion*, the stillbirths showed no macroscopic or microscopic abnormalities. Nevertheless 7 of these infants were delivered after previous toxemia. The *remaining case* was a severe thrombosis of the umbilical vein with widespread infarction of the liver.

2. Newborn Deaths between the 1st and 28th days

Newborn deaths were subdivided as follows:

1 to 24 hours of life — 2nd and 3rd days —

4th to 7th days   — 8th to 28th days.

This subdivision was an attempt to take into account the peculiarities of the perinatal and neonatal periods. PFAUNDLER (1941) states that the *metabasis*, the transfer from intrauterine to extrauterine life, "is the centre of a hazardous event, casting his shadow not only forwards but also backwards". The first three days of life — the *trihemeron* — are marked by a high mortality rate, which is considered to be an expression of unsuccessful adaptability to the extrauterine world.

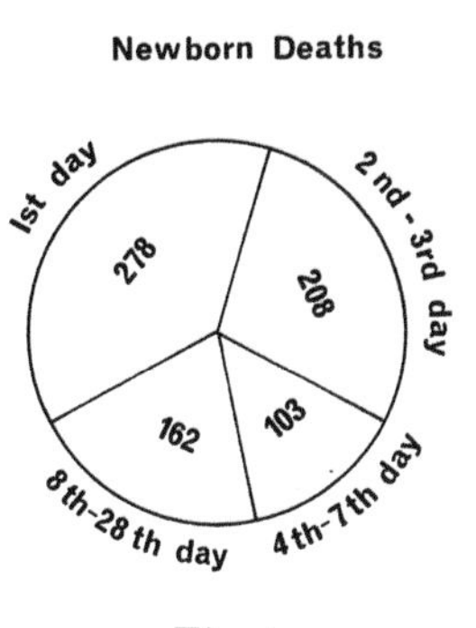

Fig. 1

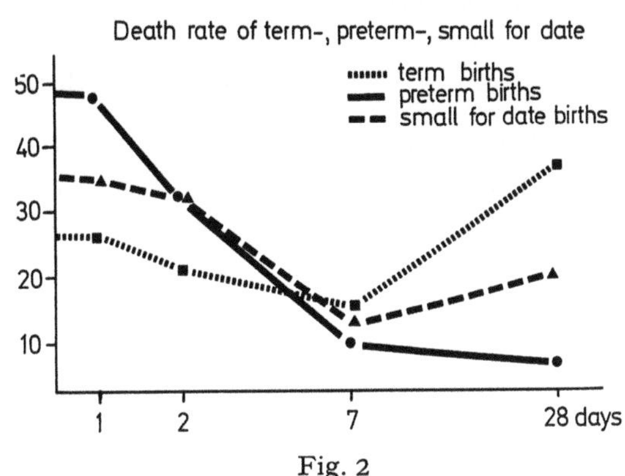

Fig. 2

Results. There were 751 newborns who died between the first hour and the 28th day. The distribution of newborn deaths is shown in Fig. 1.

One third of the newborns did not survive the first day, and two thirds died in the first three days; four fifths of the deaths occurred in the first week.

These results are in good agreement with those of other investigators. Biostatistics from the Federal Republic of Germany (1965) record a first-day mortality rate of 35 %. BUTLER and BONHAM (1963) noted a mortality rate of 45 % on the first day and of 68 % within the first three days. DHOM and KAFFARNIK (1958) recorded, 75 % of the neonatal deaths within the trihemeron.

3. Death Rate of Term, Preterm and Small-for-date Births

The death rates of the individual groups are shown in Fig. 2.

These results permit the following interpretation: Deaths of the prematurely born are closely connected with birth and with adaptation to extrauterine life. Mortality rate of term births and of small-for-date births also shows a metabasis peak. However, the mortality rate in the later neonatal period becomes increasingly high. These deaths demonstrate clearly that it is a question of *sick children* and not of difficulties in adaptation.

III. Primary Necropsy Findings

The primary cause of death is given prominence. If there is more than one significant finding, the most important is considered decisive, double registrations being purposely avoided. The analysis includes

1. Congenital malformations
2. Hemolytic diseases
3. Asphyxia
4. Respiration disturbances
5. Infections
6. Metabolic disturbances
7. Iatrogenic trauma
8. No pathological findings

1. Congenital Malformations

Cases were assigned to this category in the presence of a malformation which was considered to be incompatible with life or immediately responsible for death in the first month of life. If several functionally significant malformations were present, that representing the least chance of survival is listed as the cause of death. The malformations were categorized under the headings of organ systems.

Malformations were the primary cause of death of 235 babies (31%). Distribution according to organ system, to sex and to term, preterm and small-for-date births is shown in Table 5.

Overall, more males evidenced malformations (58%); among the cardiovascular anomalies, incidence among males reached 70%. The incidence of malformations of the central nervous system (60%) and to a lesser degree of the alimentary system was greater among females. Individual maturity groups were variously represented: term births were predominant, whilst preterm births constituted the smallest group.

Table 5. Congenital malformations: Distribution according to organ system, sex and individual maturity groups

Percent	no of cases		Organ system	no of cases		
%	♂	♀		term	preterm	small-for-date
41	67	30	Cardiovascular	76	5	16
26	29	34	Alimentary	35	6	22
15	13	22	Central nervous	19	4	12
5	7	3	Urogenital	3	2	5
10	11	12	Musculature	13	2	8
3	6	1	Pulmonary		6	1
100%	133	102		146	25	64

Cardiovascular system showed an abnormality in one fourth of all fatal malformations. The anomalies included obstruction to the outflow of the right ventricle (17), of the left ventricle (25), endocardial fibroelastosis (8), hypoplasia of the left heart (3), transposition of the great vessels (23), persistent truncus (6), septal defects combined with cor biloculare (3). The remainder (12) included severe anomalies of the pulmonary veins, ductus arteriosus and position of the heart.

Alimentary system. Esophageal atresia and tracheo-esophageal fistulae (34), atresia of the duodenum (5), of the small bowel (9), of the anus or rectum (7) and megacolon (6) were the most common anomalies. In 6 cases the esophageal atresia was associated with atresia of the duodenum (3) or of the anus (2), while one child presented all three.

Central nervous system. The most common lesion was myelomeningocele (16), anencephalus was seen in 9 cases, cyclops in 2 cases. Excessive hydrocephalus, microcephalus, defects of the brain and a sacral teratoma were the other malformations.

Urogenital system. Bilateral renal agenesis was present 5 times, hypoplasia of the kidney due to cystic degeneration 4 times and in one newborn boy (4 days) a tumor (150 gm) of the left kidney was seen.

Among the malformations of the *musculature* there were 17 cases of diaphragmatic agenesis and 6 exomphalos.

Pulmonary system was involved with cysts (3), cystic lymphangiectasis (1) and severe hypoplasia (3).

2. Hemolytic Diseases

Hemolytic diseases were the cause of death in 33 cases (4.2%). Blood group incompatibility was predominant: Rhesus incompatibility was seen in 19 cases, AB0-incompatibility in 2 and Kell-blood group incompatibility in 1. Eleven newborn babies suffered from jaundice, severe anemia, hydrops or effusion in the serous cavities, though no blood group incompatibility was observed. With the exception of one case of familial Fanconi's anemia it was impossible to determine the cause of the hemolytic diseases. The *age of the infants* was low: 31 died in the first week. Rhesus incompatibility was seen once in a first-born, 7 times in second-born, 3 times in each of a third and 4th child and once in a fifth. The exceedingly rare Kell-incompatibility was observed in the fifth child of a 29 year-old mother who had already lost her second and fourth children immediately after delivery.

3. Asphyxia

CLAIREAUX *et al.* (1960) consider the signs of pathomorphological asphyxia to be: aspiration of amniotic fluid and/or meconium, fatty degeneration of the heart, liver, and kidney, hemorrhage of the serous membranes, of the lungs or suprarenal glands, subdural, intraventricular hemorrhage and damage to the brain vessels. Division into three subgroups was useful in assessing the cause of death.

Group A. Asphyxia *without hemorrhage* and the following findings: excessive inhalation of amniotic debris and/or meconium into bronchi, alveolar ducts and alveoli, congestion of the viscera and/or hypoxemic damage of the brain.

Group B. Asphyxia *with hemorrhage* and the following findings: hemorrhage of organs, membranes, serosa, perivascular hemorrhage, congestion.

Group C. Asphyxia *with cerebral hemorrhage*. Deaths in this category showed evidence of asphyxia as described in groups A and B but in addition showed subdural, intraventricular hemorrhage and/or damage of the great cerebral veins.

Results: Asphyxia was the cause of death in 21.%. Of the 155 babies, 136 died in the first week. Distribution of the various forms within the individual maturity groups is shown in Table 6.

Table 6

Asphyxia group	No. of			
	term	preterm	small-for-date	total
A: without hemorrhage	19	7	7	33
B: with hemorrhage	9	15	11	35
C: with cerebral hemorrhage	9	66	12	87
Total	37	88	30	155

Asphyxia with cerebral hemorrhage was predominant. Schmidt (1965) stated that leptomeningeal hemorrhage is the province of the premature baby and is four times as frequent in such babies as in term births. This observation was evident in the present survey.

4. Respiratory Disturbances

The analysis includes *atelectasis* only or combined with aspiration of debris or meconium, hyaline membranes or pulmonary hemorrhage; *hyaline membranes* only or combined with pulmonary hemorrhage; *pulmonary hemorrhage; pulmonary infections*. Recently, a *pneumopathia* occurring in newborn babies treated with high concentrations of oxygen during prolonged artificial ventilation has been observed. The lesions in these lungs were caused by excessive proliferation and metaplasia of the bronchial epithelium as well as interstitial fibrosis.

Results. Respiratory disturbances were the cause of death in 25 %. Of the 196 infants, 173 died during the first week, 153 during the first three days. Table 7 shows the findings in term, preterm and small-for-date births.

Table 7. Respiratory disturbances: Various forms in term, preterm and small-for-date births

Disturbance	No. of		
	term	preterm	small-for-date
Atelectasis (only)	2	22	6
combined with aspiration	4	3	2
combined with hyaline membranes	1	21	6
combined with pulmonary hemorrhage	1	7	3
Hyaline membranes (only)	5	32	8
combined with pulmonary hemorrhage	1	7	5
Pulmonary hemorrhage	6	6	2
Pulmonary infections	14	19	7
Pneumopathia	2	3	1
Total cases	36	120	40

Atelectasis (78) and hyaline membranes (58) are the commonest respiratory disturbances. BUTLER and BONHAM (1963) consider hyaline membranes to be 8 times more frequent in premature than in term births. The present survey is in accordance with their results: 60 preterm and 7 term births. Hyaline membranes as a *primary cause of death* were estimated by v. GAVALLÉR (1959) to be 65 %, by SIVANESAN (1961) to be 47 % and by KEUTH (1965) to be 34.8 %. The present study indicates it to be 7 %, in preterm births it reaches 11 %. This falling trend may reflect the success of therapeutic endeavours. On the other hand, the *pneumopathia* indicates the dangers of therapy: According to NORTHWAY *et al.* (1967), NASH *et al.* (1967), BECKER and KOPPE (1969) and PUSEY *et al.* (1969), the structural changes in neonatal hyaline membrane disease following prolonged treatment with high concentrations of oxygen prove toxic to the lungs.

Pulmonary infections were due to staphylococci, Pseudomonas aeruginosa, coli or Klebsiella bacilli. In one female baby born in the 24th week of gestation who died 40 min after delivery, a widespread giant cell pneumonia with numerous multinuclear giant cells was seen (MOLZ, 1971).

5. Infections

Extrapulmonary (18) and generalized (57) infections were the cause of death in 10 %. Bacterial infections (65) were predominant. The causative organism was detected in 53 cases: half were due to staphylococci (27), 9, to Pseudomonas aeruginosa and Escherichia coli, 5, to listeria one each to meningo-and pneumococci. *Tuberculosepsis* with numerous caseous and hard tubercles in the intestinal organs, lungs, brain, bone marrow, endocrine organs and spermatic cord was seen in a 21-day-old boy. In 12 other cases treated with antibiotics no causative organism was determined. The remaining cases included: lues connata (3), cytomegalic inclusion disease (3), hepatitis epidemica (1), viral myocarditis (1) and candidiasis (1); the etiology of a granulomatous lesions in the brain of a 4 day-old-child is unknown.

6. Metabolic Disturbances

Metabolic diseases were the cause of death in 24 babies (3 %). The diseases included metabolic inborn errors such as galactosemia (1), valin-leucinemia (1), hereditary epidermolysis bullosa (1) and mucoviscidosis (5). The other cases included fetopathia diabetica (9), chondrodystrophia and osteogenesis imperfecta (2 of each), arthrogryposis congenita (1) and 2 cases with severe acetonemia. The lesions in one of these children were unusual: a 3-hour-old male newborn, whose mother suffered from uremia, showed papillary necrosis of the kidney, ulcerative cystitis, severe anemia and pulmonary edema.

7. Iatrogenic Trauma

Ten babies suffered from birth traumas—fractures of the skull, lesions of the brain and spine, rupture of the liver. Two babies died from hemopericardium following penetrating wounds due to the catheterization of the heart in one other child the portal vein was ruptured by the catheter.

8. No Pathological Findings

No primary necropsy findings could be found in 2 term and 18 preterm births. Disorders in the mother were ascertained in 6 preterm births: placenta praevia, placental fibrosis, infiltration of the decidua and premature rupture (–6 days) of the membranes. One of the term births suffered from Turner's syndrome; the second child died suddenly on the 28th day.

IV. Cause of Death in Term, Preterm and Small-for-Date Births

Malformations, hemolytic diseases, asphyxia, respiratory disturbances and infections predominated in each group which together comprised, 90 % or more. Divergence in *incidence* of the various causes of death is, however, clearly seen in Fig. 3.

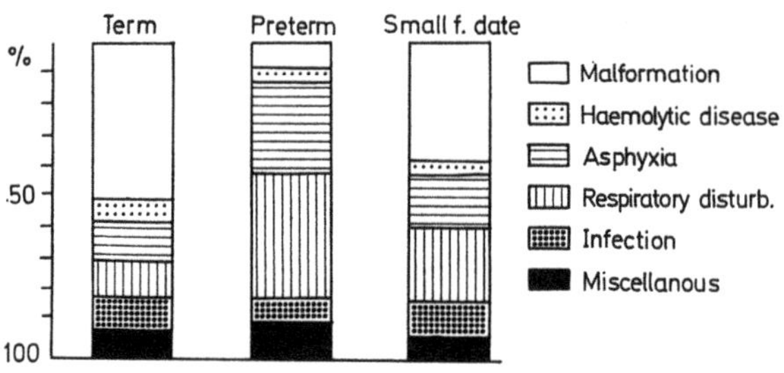

Fig. 3

Cause of death	Term	Preterm	Small-for-date
Malformations	51 %	8.4 %	38 %
Hemolytic diseases	6	4	3.5
Asphyxia	13	30	18
Respiratory disturbances	13	40	24
Infections	11	8	13
Metabolic disturbances	3.5	2.6	3
Iatrogenic trauma	2.5	1	(1)
No pathological findings	(2)	6	—

It may be seen from the results that the *preterm births* represent a group in themselves, whereas the *term births* and *small-for-date births* are an inherently related group: in preterm births respiratory distress and asphyxia constitute 70%. These predominant causes of death are clear evidence of the failure of these babies to adapt to the demands of extrauterine life. In term and small-for-date births malformations head the list these babies are not viable owing to some defect in development.

V. Causes of Death in the Perinatal and Later Neonatal Periods

Table 8 contains a comparison of the primary findings from necropsies performed on babies who died during the perinatal and later neonatal periods.

Table 8. Cause of death in the perinatal and later neonatal periods

0–7 days		Cause of death	8–28 days	
no. of cases	%		%	no. of cases
162	22.7	Malformations	52.4	84
50	7.0	Hemolytic diseases	1.2	2
210	29.4	Asphyxia	4.9	8
173	24.2	Respiratory disturbances	14.2	23
45	6.3	Infections	19.7	32
17	2.3	Metabolic disturbances	6.1	10
13	1.8	Iatrogenic trauma	1.2	2
1	0.1	Remainder		
41	5.7	No pathological findings	0.6	1
712				162

It is evident that of the *perinatal deaths* every third is due to asphyxia and every fourth to respiratory distress. However, malformations were responsible for the death of every fifth child. In the *later neonatal period* every second child died of a congenital malformation and every fifth of general infection; pulmonary infections were responsible for the death of every seventh child.

C. Subdivision B: Multiple Births

Among the 970 cases, there were 94 twins and 2 triplets —9.9%. This result is in accordance with the incidence reported by BUTLER and BONHAM (1963) who found 10.1% multiple births among 7117 deaths.

Preterm births (76 = 80%) were predominant, whereas *term births* (8) and *small-for-date births* (12) were small groups. There are 56 males and 40 females. Of the 94 twins, 40 were twin A and 54 twin B; 46 twins were twin-pairs. In 5 other cases the twin partner also died but was not autopsied. Twin A only succumbed 15 times and twin B only 28 times. An overall excess of twin B deaths is indicated by BUTLER and ALBERMAN (1969) who found 410 deaths amoung twin B as against 295 among twin A. BACH and KIEFE (1962) reported the neonatal mortality proportion of twin A to twin B as 11.4% to 18%; KEUTH et al. (1964), as 17.9% against 25.5% in the cases of preterm twin births.

Of the triplets one is triplet B, the other triplet C.

The *order of birth*, known in 90 cases, is presented in Table 9.

Table 9. Order of births among twins and triplets

Order of birth	Twin A	Twin B	Triplet B	Triplet C
1	28			
2	4	34	1	
3		5		
4	2	5		
5	1	3		
6	1	3		
7		1		1
15	1			
All cases	37	51	1	1

Breech presentations (23) and *abnormal position* (10) were seen in every third twin. Twin B (26) was affected approximately 4 times more frequently than twin A. Obstetrical intervention was necessary with every second child. Among the vertex presentations there are 3 twin A, with assisted deliveries. The *7 stillbirths* including 2 twin-pairs, 2 twin B and 1 twin A. The primary necropsy findings are summarized in Table 10.

Table 10. Primary necropsy findings in twin A and twin B

Twin A			Necropsy findings	Twin B		
term	preterm	small-for-date		small-for-date	preterm	term
1	2	2	Malformations	1	1	1
1	11	1	Asphyxia	1	12	
1	12	2	Respiratory disturbances	1	23	3
1	3		Infections		6	
	2		Trauma	1	2	
			Remainder	1		
		1	No pathological findings	1		
4	30	6		6	44	4

The *malformations* involved the alimentary system (4), nervous system (3) and the musculature (1).

The distribution of the various forms of *asphyxia* included: *group A*, 7 cases, *group B*, 4 cases and *group C*, 15 cases.

Of the 40 *respiratory disturbances, atelectasis occurred only* in 13 cases, combined *with aspiration* in 4, *with hyaline membranes* in 6 and *hemorrhage* in 1. *Hyaline membranes only* were seen in 8 cases and combined with hemorrhage in 1. Massive *pulmonary hemorrhage* was observed in 2 cases, *pulmonary infections* in 4 and *pneumopathia* in 1.

Extrapulmonary infections were due to staphylococci (4), *Escherichia coli* (4), Pseudomonas aeruginosa (1) and streptococci (1).

Three twin B's suffered from *traumatic damage* of the liver or thoracic organs caused by twin A during labor. Rupture of the liver was sustained by one twin A during manual extraction in breech presentation. The remaining case was an encephalomalacia of unknown etiology. No pathological findings could be detected in two small-for-date births. Both triplets suffered from respiratory disturbances.

D. Conclusions

Postmortem studies represent a random selection of all deaths occurring during the perinatal and newborn periods. The results therefore allow conclusions to be drawn about perinatal mortality and risks to newborns. In the present study, assessment of the results indicates the following:
— consistently high incidence of first-born children in the individual maturity groups
— overall excess of twin B deaths
— higher mortality for males in preterm and term births with a maximum at birth weights of over 4000 gm
— preponderance of males among cases of fatal malformations, with a maximum in cardiovascular lesions
— preponderance of females among cases of malformation of the central nervous system
— abnormal presentation among every second child in twins, every fifth in preterm and every tenth in term and small-for-date
— assisted deliveries among term births in approximately every fifth child, among preterm and small-for-date births, in every tenth child
— of the stillbirths, half of the deaths were due to asphyxia; every second child died at the end of gestation and antepartum
— term and small-for-date births differ from preterm in their lower transitional and rising mortality rate in the later neonatal period
— fatal malformations take first place among causes of death of term and small-for-date births; in preterm births respiratory disturbances are predominant.
— preterm births were subject to alveolar hyaline membranes 6 times as frequently as term births and 3 times more frequently than small-for-date births
— cerebral hemorrhage with asphyxia was 4 times more frequent in preterm births

E. Summary

Autopsies were performed by the same pathologist using a standard technique on 130 stillbirths and 840 newborn deaths. The infants are divided according to single or multiple births.

The ratio of term, preterm and small-for-date births against perinatal and newborn mortality is examined. Higher mortality rates among first-born children as well as extremely high mortality rates during the first three days of life are characteristic of every group. In the perinatal period asphyxia and respiratory disturbances are the most frequent cause of death. Fatal malformations take first place among the causes of death of term and small-for-date births in the later neonatal period.

References

Bach, H. G., Kiefe, M.: Die Zwillingsgeburten an der Universitäts-Frauenklinik Heidelberg 1950–1959. Arch. Gynäk. 196, 609 (1962).

Becker, M. J., Koppe, J. G.: Pulmonary structural changes in neonatal hyaline membrane disease treated with high pressure artificial respiration. Thorax 24, 689 (1969).

Bretscher, J.: Der klinische Aspekt von 1061 perinatal verstorbenen Kindern. Arch. Gynäk. 204, 107 (1967).

Butler, N. R., Alberman, E. D.: Perinatal problems. The second report of the 1958 British Perinatal Mortality Survey. Edinburgh—London: E. & S. Livingstone LTD 1969.

Butler, N. R., Bonham, D. G.: Perinatal mortality. The first report of the 1958 British Perinatal Mortality Survey. Edinburgh—London: E. & S. Livingstone LTD 1963.

Claireaux, A. E.: Perinatal mortality in the United Kingdom. Modern trends in obstetrics 3rd chaptre 13, 191. London: Butterworths 1963.

Claireaux, A. E., Fraser, A. C., Marshall, W. C.: Some observations on anoxia as a cause of death in the foetus and newborn. J. Obstet. Gynaec. Brit. Emp. 67, 763 (1960).

Davis, J. A., Payne, W. W., Stevens, J., Yu, J.: Some metabolic aspects of the ill premature infant with the respiratory distress syndrome. Helv. paediat. Acta 24, 609 (1969).

Dhom, G., Kaffarnik, H.: Sektionsstatistische Untersuchungen zur Neugeborenen- und Säuglingssterblichkeit. Öff. Gesundh.-Dienst 19, 515 (1958).

Gavallér, B. v.: Die hyalinen Membranen in den Lungen Neugeborener. Verh. dtsch. Ges. Path. 43, 195 (1959).

Keuth, U.: Das Membransyndrom der Früh- und Neugeborenen. Exp. Med., Pathol. u. Klinik, Band 16. Berlin—Heidelberg—New York: Springer 1965.

Keuth, U., Schmidt, E., Tzieply, G., Widtman, V.: Untersuchungen zur unterschiedlichen perinatalen Schädigung von Zwillingen. Z. Kinderheilk. 91, 265 (1964).

Kolb, G.: Todesursachen in der ersten Lebenswoche. Z. ärztl. Fortbild. 53, 136 (1964).

Molz, G.: Pränatale Pneumonie mit mehrkernigen Riesenzellen bei einem immaturen Frühgeborenen. Helv. paediat. Acta 26, 593 (1971).

Morf, E.: Die pathologisch-anatomischen Hauptbefunde bei 1061 perinatal verstorbenen Kindern. Inaugural Dissertation Zürich 1966.

Mütter- und Säuglingssterblichkeit in der Bundesrepublik Deutschland. Referat Dtsch. med. Wschr. 90, 1378 (1965).

Nash, G., Blennerhasset, J. B., Pontoppidan, H.: Pulmonary lesions associated with oxygen therapy and arteficial ventilation. New Engl. J. Med. 276, 368 (1967).

Nesbitt, R. E. L., Anderson, W.: Perinatal mortality. Clinical and pathologic aspects. Obstet. and Gynec. 8, 60 (1956).

Neuweiler, W., Lutziger, H.: Die perinatale Mortalität an der Frauenklinik Bern von 1947–1964. Vortrag Jahresversammlung Schweiz. Ges. Pädiatrie Lugano 1966.

Northway, W. H., Rosan, R. C., Porter, D. Y.: Pulmonary disease following prolonged therapy of hyaline-membrane disease. New Engl. J. Med. 276, 357 (1967).

Pfaundler, M.: Studien über Frühtod, Geschlechtsverhältnis und Selektion. Z. Kinderheilk. 62, 351 (1941).

Pfaundler, M.: In: Keller, W., Wiskott, A.: Lehrbuch der Kinderheilkunde, S. 52. Stuttgart: Georg Thieme 1961.

Pusey, V. A., MacPherson, R. I., Chernick, V.: Pulmonary fibroplasia following prolonged artificial ventilation of newborn infants. Canad. med. Ass. J. 100, 451 (1969).

Schmidt, H.: Untersuchungen zur Pathogenese und Aetiologie der geburtstraumatischen Hirnschädigungen Früh- und Reifgeborener. Veröffentl. morph. Pathol. Heft 70. Stuttgart: Gustav Fischer 1965.

Sivanesan, S.: Neonatal pulmonary pathology in Singapore. J. Pediat. 59, 600 (1961).

Westergaard; In: Pfaundler, M. Studien über Frühtod, Geschlechtsverhältnis und Selektion. Z. Kinderheilk. 62, 351 (1941).

Zschoch, H., Mahnke, P. F.: Die pathologische Anatomie des Kindesalters in der Sektionsstatistik. Jena: VEB Gustav Fischer Verlag 1968.

Subject Index

The numbers set in *italics* refer to those pages on which the respective catch-word is discussed in detail

Index to Volumes 37—57

Ergebnisse der allgemeinen Pathologie und der pathologischen Anatomie

Current Topics in Pathology

Current Topics in Pathology

Ergebnisse der Pathologie

Reprint from

Vol. 58

Experimental Metabolic Disorders and the Subcellular Reaction Pattern

H. P. Rohr, U. N. Riede

With 25 Figures

Springer-Verlag Berlin · Heidelberg · New York 1973

Current Topics in
Pathology

Ergebnisse der Pathologie

Reprint from

Vol. 58

Insulitis - A Morphological Review

G. Freytag, G. Klöppel

With 18 Figures

Springer-Verlag Berlin · Heidelberg · New York 1973

Current Topics in Pathology

Ergebnisse der Pathologie

Reprint from

Vol. 58

Printed in Germany

Cytologic and Histologic Aspects
of Toxically Induced Liver Reactions

O. Klinge

With 8 Figures

Springer-Verlag Berlin · Heidelberg · New York 1973

Current Topics in
Pathology

Ergebnisse der Pathologie

Reprint from Vol. 58

Printed in Germany

Age-Related Bone Changes

G. Delling

With 15 Figures

Springer-Verlag Berlin · Heidelberg · New York 1973

Current Topics in Pathology

Ergebnisse der Pathologie

Vol. 58

Perinatal and Newborn Deaths

G. Molz

With 3 Figures

Springer-Verlag Berlin · Heidelberg · New York 1973

R. Burkhardt

Bone Marrow and Bone Tissue

Color Atlas of Clinical Histopathology

By **Rolf Burkhardt,**
Dr. med., apl. Professor an
der Universität München
With a Foreword by
Professor Dr. **Walther Stich**
Translated by
Dr. **H. J. Hirsch,** London

With 721 colored figures
XII, 115 pages
Format: $12^{1}/_{2} \times 11^{1}/_{2}''$. 1971
Cloth DM 248,—; US $101.70

Thanks to the evolution
of new biopsy and
histological preparation
methods—a development
to which the author has
substantially contributed—it
is now possible
to illustrate the normal and
pathological histology
of bone and bone marrow
in a more detailed and
informative manner
than heretofore possible.
The atlas provides a morphological documentation
of the potential applications
of this new approach
in clinical practice and
fundamental research.
More than 700 colored
photomicrographs were
selected from a series of some
2000 myelotomies of the
human pelvis.
They provide convincing
evidence that the histobiopsy
method is superior
to sternal puncture and
cytological smears for the
study and interpretation of

pathological changes
in the bone marrow.
This applies equally to the
study of blood diseases
proper and the role played
by bone marrow in other
types of diseases.
Undoubtedly this work will
contribute to a reevaluation
of the clinical and
morphological diagnostic
procedures used for
an organ that is involved
in so many vital
pathobiological processes.

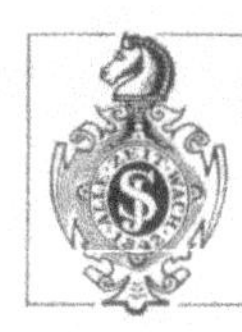

**Springer-Verlag
Berlin
Heidelberg
New York**

München Johannesburg
London New Delhi Paris
Rio de Janeiro Sydney
Tokyo Wien

www.ingramcontent.com/pod-product-compliance
Ingram Content Group UK Ltd.
Pitfield, Milton Keynes, MK11 3LW, UK
UKHW052347070726
473059UK00009B/2581